research:

THE VALIDATION OF CLINICAL PRACTICE

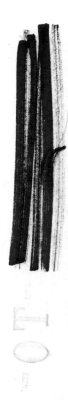

research:
THE VALIDATION OF CLINICAL PRACTICE

Otto D. Payton, Ph.D.
Professor and Director of Graduate Studies in Physical Therapy
School of Allied Health Professions
Medical College of Virginia
Virginia Commonwealth University
Richmond, Virginia

 F. A. DAVIS COMPANY / Philadelphia

Library of Congress Cataloging in Publication Data

Payton, Otto D.
   Research: the validation of clinical practice.

   Includes bibliographies and index.
   1. Physical therapy—Research.   2. Occupational
therapy—Research.   3. Medical research.   I. Title.
RM708.P38   615'.82   78-26362
ISBN 0-8036-6798-1

TO MARY, COLLEEN, AND SUE

FOREWORD

In Chapter 1 the author makes several forceful statements about the role of research in the development of scientific knowledge and the adaptation of this knowledge in the clinical setting. He is correct in pointing out that practitioners in the fields of occupational and physical therapy must cultivate research skills, and, accordingly, faculties must be prepared to teach them.

Research methods can be presented in a variety of ways. This text deals with practical applications at the introductory level, and is intended specifically for students on their way to becoming occupational and physical therapists and for practicing clinicians who did not have this information in their basic preparation program. The writer of the book does not imply that research methodology for physical therapists and occupational therapists is any different from that of any other practitioner; this text, however, will be most helpful to students enrolled in occupational and physical therapy programs since the examples used deal with these fields.

This book is certainly needed at this point in the evolution of these two professions. The material is presented in a manner which should encourage students to learn methodology and to apply new skills.

Thomas C. Barker, Ph.D.
Dean, School of Allied Health Professions
Medical College of Virginia
Past President, American Society
of Allied Health Professions

INTRODUCTION

The purpose of this book is to provide a basic text which examines and explains the process by which we can test and improve what we do, as health professionals, to and for patients. The intended audience is undergraduate students and practicing clinicians in the fields of occupational therapy and physical therapy. As future health professionals they should be prepared to defend, with rational and scientific evidence, the appropriateness and effectiveness (i.e., the validity) of their practice and procedures. In order to do that they must be able to read (or hear) the scientific statements of other professionals, interpret them correctly, and incorporate them into their own practice. To some will come the incentive and the opportunity to contribute to that body of knowledge which supports and sustains their practice. What I am talking about, of course, is research, a word much maligned and unreasonably feared by some people. All the word research really means is a systematic search for reliable knowledge. Most of this book will be about reading and interpreting the research of others. However, accurate research reading skills are necessary prerequisites to later performance skills.

There are five basic principles which form the foundation for this text.

1. Research is important to therapy because it is the major tool available to us for validating our services to people in our role as therapists. Although most of these people are patients, we should also include students and coworkers with whom we interact as therapists.

2. A model of therapeutic practice is useful in looking at what we know now, and what we need to know, in order to substantiate what we do as therapists.

3. Using research effectively as a tool for understanding is a skill that can be learned. There are two corollaries to this principle: (a) to become skillful in reading or doing research, one needs concepts, principles, and practice and (b) among these important concepts and principles are some related to measurement and to the scope and limitations of different research designs.

4. Validity and reliability are special characteristics which are important to measurement and to research design.

5. Theories and models are better guides to knowledge than trial and error.

This text takes a nonmathematical approach. It will attempt to give the reader those concepts with which scientific literature can be read and understood, including the *meaning* of statistics and how they may be interpreted for practical use. Some of the information in this book will also lay the foundation for selecting statistical tools. Should the reader choose to pursue that topic further at a later date, the formulas and their calculations may be sought in the references provided. The writing of scientific reports will not be dealt with extensively, but references to other resources will be given.

The concepts and principles presented in the text will be illustrated with several relevant reprints from the literature of occupational therapy, physical therapy, and related fields. These reprints, located at the end of the book, will be used throughout the text to examine, analyze, and exemplify the concepts being developed and will give the student an opportunity to check his understanding of the textual material. Only articles which can be presented in positive and complementary ways were chosen.

The question may be posed as to whether students and practitioners in the allied health professions need the kind of knowledge and skills dealt with in this text. The *Standards for Physical Therapy Services*, adopted by the Board of Directors of the American Physical Therapy Association[1] as a self-evaluation guide, states in Article XI:

The Physical Therapy Service conducts or participates in research projects that may contribute knowledge for improved patient care and for the growth of physical therapy as a profession . . . . The type and extent of research projects will be determined by the qualifications of the staff and the availability of facilities, equipment, and finances. The staff members are encouraged to publish the results of their investigations.

A companion document entitled *Standards for the Physical Therapy Practitioner*,[2] adopted by the House of Delegates of the American Physical Therapy Association in June 1975 for self-assessment of the individual therapist, states in Article VII:

> The physical therapist understands the significance of research and, when possible, participates in research activities .... The physical therapist recognizes research as an integral part of the profession of physical therapy, supports and assists those engaged in research, and has a basic understanding of the interpretation of research studies. The physical therapist conducting research has a sufficient knowledge of research principles and methodology.

It seems clear, then, that the practitioner and the physical therapy student needs certain fundamental skills in understanding research and interpreting research studies. They are also strongly encouraged, wherever possible, to participate in research activities. According to a recent report by Currier,[3] in September 1976, all but 2 of the 71 approved basic programs in physical therapy had some form of didactic instruction in research; 73 percent had a separate course, and 77 percent of these courses were taught by the physical therapy faculty. The average for the 69 schools was 24 hours of instruction. Seventy-eight percent of courses included some statistics, but the emphasis was on interpretation. Fifty-six percent of these schools used a textbook, but all texts used were from outside the field of physical therapy. Thus the need for a text such as this becomes clear.

A similar story may be told for the discipline of occupational therapy. In their *Guide for Graduate Education in Occupational Therapy Leading to the Master's Degree*,[4] the following statement may be found:

> The graduate of a master's program in occupational therapy has beginning competencies in scientific inquiry, methodologies, and scholarly writing and is able to apply these competencies to the development of occupational therapy theory, and practice.

Likewise, the *Essentials of an Accredited Educational Program for the Occupational Therapist*,[5] under Section G: Curriculum, states that upon completion of the course of study the student shall be able to

> promote, plan, implement, and conduct research for the benefit of the public and the growth of the profession.

"Principles of Research" are cited as possible content resources for the implementation of the basic professional program.

Objectives at the beginning of each chapter are provided to alert the reader to competencies which they could acquire as a result of studying and working with that chapter. At the end of each chapter, questions are provided which the reader may use for self-assessment of subject matter mastery.

The teacher may wish to make supplemental reading assignments in appropriate literature in order to give students more practice in identifying key concepts and principles, in addition to the articles reprinted at the back of the book. A useful instructional-learning strategy is to use a journal club format in which the participants report on current journal articles of interest, emphasizing the question asked, the research design, methods of data treatment, interpretation and results, and the compatibility of the various elements in the research project. Such a journal club could also be used by clinicians in their inservice programs to develop skill in critical reading. Independent readers may simply work on their own to develop the same skills as they read.

Rather than use the traditional masculine gender as representing both sexes or the awkward he/she, his/her notations, I have elected to use both masculine and feminine genders indiscriminately in this text. In this way the text may be more reflective of real life and not of a particular bias.

Acknowledgment of intellectual indebtedness is an impossible task. So many people have influenced and informed my thinking that a list will not be attempted. Special recognition should be made of the students who, over the last seven years, have listened to the spoken version of this book in class and helped to clarify ideas and methods of presentation. Last, but not least, special credit should be given to my wife, Mary, and my secretary, Ava Street, who patiently typed the original draft, the revisions, and the final copy of this manuscript.

REFERENCES

1. American Physical Therapy Association: *Standards for physical therapy services.* Physical Therapy 51:1315–1318, 1971.
2. *Standards for the Physical Therapy Practitioner.* American Physical Therapy Association, Washington, D.C., 1975.
3. Currier, D.: *Research patterns for basic physical therapy education.* Paper presented to the Section on Research, American Physical Therapy Association, Combined Sections Meeting, Phoenix, Arizona, February 1977.
4. *Guide for Graduate Education in Occupational Therapy Leading to the Master's Degree.* Council on Education, American Occupational Therapy Association, Washington, D.C., 1976.

5. *Essentials of an Accredited Educational Program for the Occupational Therapist.* American Occupational Therapy Association, Washington, D.C., 1973.

CONTENTS

Chapter 1

BASIC CONCEPTS IN RESEARCH

OBJECTIVES

1. *Discuss role of research in professional development.*
2. *Discuss four ways of knowing.*
3. *Define and illustrate: research, concept, principle, data, statistics, hypothesis.*
4. *Define and illustrate goals and purposes of research.*
5. *Outline scientific method.*
6. *Identify the purpose and question in a given research report.*
7. *Define several research questions based on one goal; state null and alternate hypotheses.*
8. *State several typical assumptions underlying many clinical research problems; identify assumptions in given literature.*
9. *Define primary and secondary sources; list several common fallacies in citing authorities.*

ROLE OF RESEARCH

Research should begin with an intellectual itch which needs scratching. The "itch" is a question for which you need an answer not immediately available. You may want to know the answer to that question out of purely intellectual curiosity, or you may want the

1

answer because you need it in order to solve a clinical or professional problem. The "scratching" is the answer to the question in the form of reliable facts, concepts, or principles which may be used either to generate more complex principles or to assist in solving a practical problem. For example, you might need to know why some patients in a given disease category respond well to a treatment procedure while other patients who are apparently comparable do not respond well to the same procedure. You want this information in order to improve the quality of care in your clinic.

These kinds of questions can only be answered by practicing clinicians or by people who are looking over the shoulder of the clinician in order to learn about clinical practice. If your chosen profession is to remain independent, but at the same time to grow and maintain a reputable position in the health care system, then an understanding and appreciation of the role of the research is necessary. A widespread responsibility on the part of all professional practitioners should be to make some contribution, in some way, to the scientific validation of their practice; that means research—the discovery and validation of the concepts and principles on which practice is based. The research mentality (and it is as much as state of mind as it is a process) should be an everyday working tool of the practitioner. In the words of Pruden,[1] we need to strip research of its "aura of glamour or mystery, to reduce it to a size that fits our laboratory workbench, and to make it a realistic part of each of our daily activities."

WAYS OF KNOWING

How does one "know" something? How does one know that a given fact is so? How does one know that a given procedure tests what it is supposed to test, that it works every time and is dependable? How does one know the causes of certain patient reactions to therapeutic interventions? In other words, what are the sources of reliable knowledge?

Dickoff and James[2] have defined four major ways in which people arrive at knowledge; these are modified from an original formulation by the philosopher Charles Peirce.

The first way is tenacity, or <u>intuition</u>. This method has been used by man since the beginning of human life. Unfortunately, this method may sometimes spill over into clinical practice, and the clinician will say "I know this is so simply because I know it" or ". . . because everybody knows it." There is an important place in human knowing for intuition and it has an important role to play in the scientific

2

method. Intuition should help one to define the question, and provide clues as to where answers may be found; it is not an appropriate method for validating the answer.

The second way of knowing is the way of authority, "I know that this is so because _____ (some authority) said so." In the past, authorities have said that the earth was flat; it may well be that some of today's authorities are making equally erroneous statements. If the authority figure has used tenacity, some other authority, or pure reason as the basis for his pronouncements, he may be just as erroneous as anyone. On the other hand, authorities in the field are frequently right and can be a good source of information. However, where important or highly complex questions are involved, it is best to check out the basis of "authoritative" statements.

The third way of knowing is often called the *a priori* method which means the use of reason alone, without experimental evidence. It is the method of an armchair philosopher. Reason is an extremely useful tool; it has helped mankind to achieve great things. But reason is only a tool, and how it is used makes a great deal of difference. If one applies the rules of logic to abstract ideas and verbalizations without ever checking them against concrete realities, one can easily fall into error. An excellent example of this, as well as an example of the abuse of authority, is the work of Galen. His dogmatic textbook on medicine became the medical "bible" of the Middle Ages. Because it was not based on observation, it contained more errors than it should have even in that age. Unfortunately, it supplanted the writings of Hippocrates, whose work was based on direct observation of the phenomena he discussed.

A fourth way of knowing is that combination of methods and procedures which has come to be known as "the scientific method." The scientific method has a place for intuition as a guide to what the really important questions are and where one might best look for the answer; it has a place for authority which tells us what has already been discovered by valid and reliable means; and it has a place for reason in abstracting concepts and principles from observed data. Reason is essential for interpreting what the facts mean and how they might best be used in the solution of practical problems. To these three the scientific method adds something else which is equally important, and that is observation. The direct or, if necessary, indirect observation of some aspect of reality and the careful recording of what is observed are important elements in the scientific process which has created the technology which supports our present world. The scientific method is outlined in more detail later on in this chapter, but first let us look at some basic definitions.

3

DEFINITIONS

Research is the process of looking for a specific answer to a specific question in an organized, objective, reliable way. To phrase it another way, it is a method for fixating a belief or settling an issue to a point of stability adequate for action.[2] It is goal-directed and usually action-oriented. Health science research, be it in physical therapy, occupational therapy, or some other discipline, is directed towards the development of an organized body of valid and reliable knowledge about the events of concern to the health scientist. For the clinician, the behavior of patients, particularly those behaviors which are influenced through the therapeutic process, are of central importance. The purpose of gathering this scientific body of knowledge is to enable the clinician to determine which conditions produce desirable reactions in patients.

A *concept* is an abstract idea generalized from particular instances. One has a concept of a phenomenon when one is familiar enough with its essential features that new examples of that same phenomenon can be recognized and classified wherever they are seen. The essence of concept formation is the ability to disregard the nonessential differences and pay attention to the essential characteristics of an item in order to classify it. For example, one has a concept of what a patella is if one can correctly classify all given examples, whether it be in an anatomical preparation, in a child, in an adult, in a fat person, in a thin person, etc., and whether it is whole or broken into two pieces. In each instance the individual can disregard the nonessential differences and say: this is a bone which is classified as a patella.

A *principle* states a relationship between two or more concepts. For example, if one has the concepts "patellar bone," "tendon," "quadriceps muscle," and a concept of what the word "embedded" means, then one is in a position to understand the principle that the patellar bone is embedded in the tendon of the quadriceps muscle. It would be incorrect to say that the quadriceps muscle is embedded in the tendon of the patellar bone; that is a completely different relationship. This expression of a correct relationship is also called a rule, or a generalization, or sometimes even a law.

The goal of research is to develop concepts and principles which are based on observed facts and to establish these concepts and principles to the point where they are useful for predicting future events. To give a simple example, Newton's first law is a principle which states, in part, that a body at rest will remain at rest unless some force acts to move it. Based on that principle we can predict that if you rest a coffee cup carefully on the desk in front of you, it will stay there until

4

something is done to move it. The cup will not unpredictably go wandering across the top of the desk or into your lap. In similar ways we can use concepts and principles to predict the behavior of patients in the clinical setting, and that is the ultimate goal of clinical research.

Data are special kinds of facts used in the scientific process (note that "data" is plural; its singular form is "datum"). When a therapist observes: "depressed patients are quiet," this statement is not a fact in the scientific sense, and thus is not a datum. We cannot tell from the statement whether it is based on direct observation of one person or an opinion gathered from reading. We do not know under what circumstances the observation was made and there is no indication of the possible exceptions. Are there any depressed patients who are not quiet under certain circumstances? However, if that same therapist records the observation that when Mrs. Smith was observed unobtrusively for 10 minutes while she was in a group of people who were talking to each other and Mrs. Smith was quiet throughout the 10-minute period, that is a datum. If the same kind of observation is recorded in the same way under the same circumstances for 20 different people who were diagnosed as depressed and 18 of them were quiet and 2 joined in the conversation, we now have data—20 recorded observations—upon which to make a generalization. (It may not be enough data to make a good generalization, but that is not the point here.) We might now make the generalization that, based on this limited data, 80 percent of the people who are diagnosed as depressed are quiet, where "quiet" is defined as not taking part in a conversation in a social situation. On the basis of that generalization, we might make a prediction that 80 percent of the next sample of 20 depressed people who are observed will be quiet under similar circumstances. Prediction is the ultimate goal of most scientific inquiry.

At this point the reader should be able to discern a progression from (1)the collection of data based on controlled observations of the facts in specific situations, to (2)the formulation of concepts and principles, to (3)the prediction of future events based on the generalization. Early in the process the prediction is stated in the form of a *hypothesis*. A hypothesis is simply a statement of what one would expect to occur on the basis of given data. Hypotheses are often stated in an if/then format: *if* Newton's first law is correct, *then* the cup resting on my desk will remain in that position until some force is applied to it. Another example: *if* high SAT scores are associated with success in college, *then* the students in a given program with high SAT scores will have high GPAs. A hypothesis may also be viewed as a statement of expectation based on the principles which have been formulated on the basis of the data which have been observed.

5

At this point it might be well to differentiate between goal, purpose, and hypothesis in scientific inquiry. A *goal* is a general, comprehensive statement of intention; *purpose* is more specific; *hypothesis* is most specific. For example, one might have as a goal the improvement of the functional abilities of the upper extremities of brain-damaged patients. One of many related purposes might be to test the validity of the Rood method of treatment for facilitating control of the upper extremities. One of many hypotheses related to that one purpose might be that if extensor tone is increased through stimulation of the tonic labyrinthine reflex and through vibration of extensor musculature, then spastic children with cerebral palsy who fulfill certain criteria should have more functional use of their elbow extensors after vibration of the triceps in the inverted position.

One last definition: a *statistic* is a numerical statement about a group of observations. It is a mathematical tool which serves two purposes: (1)summarizing data, and (2)making a mathematical statement of the confidence which you can place in a particular principle, generalization, or hypothesis. In other words, statistics are mathematical ways of summarizing data and of telling you the chances of being right and the chances of being wrong when you make a prediction based on the summarized data. The interpretation of statistical information is dealt with more fully in Chapter 3.

THE SCIENTIFIC METHOD

Some writers would contend that there is no such thing as the scientific method. This is true in the sense that different scientists put their individual stamp on what they do, and it is true that they do not necessarily follow a rigid set of procedures, step by step. In fact, most researchers bounce back and forth from one step to another in every conceivable sequence in their efforts to answer questions about their research interest. However, it is also true that there is a generally recognized pattern which is inherent in most scientific endeavors. This section presents a generalized pattern of the scientific approach to problem-solving.

Assumptions of the Scientific Method

Before we look at that pattern itself let us look at some of the assumptions underlying the scientific method. Most scientists do not give these assumptions a great deal of thought from day to day, and that is why they are called assumptions. Nevertheless, they are the basis of the researchers' daily activities in the same way that a founda-

6

tion supports a building. The clearest statement of these assumptions that I know of was made by Dressel and Mayhew[3] in a 1954 study sponsored by the American Council on Education:

1. *Principle of Objectivity:* A scientist cultivates the ability to examine facts and suspend judgment with regard to his observations, conclusions, and activities.

2. *Principle of Consistency:* A scientist assumes that the behavior of the universe is not capricious, but is describable in terms of consistent laws, such that when two sets of conditions are the same, the same consequences may be expected.

3. *Principle of Tentativeness:* A scientist does not regard his generalizations as final, but is willing to modify them if they are contradicted by new evidence.

4. *Principle of Causality:* A scientist believes that every phenomenon results from a discoverable cause.

5. *Principle of Uniformity:* A scientist believes that the forces which are now operating in the world are those which have always operated, and that the world and the universe which we see are the result of their continuous operation.

6. *Principle of Simplicity:* A scientist prefers simple and widely applicable explanations of phenomena. He attempts to reduce his view of the world to as simple terms as possible.

7. *Principle of Materiality:* A scientist prefers material and mechanical explanations of phenomena, rather than those which depend on nonmaterial and supernatural forces.

8. *Principle of Dynamism:* A scientist expects nature to be dynamic rather than static, and to show variation and change.

9. *Principle of Relativeness:* A scientist thinks of the world and of things in it, as sets of relationships rather than as absolutes.

10. *Principle of Intergradation:* A scientist thinks in terms of continua; he distrusts sharp boundary lines, and expects to find related classes of natural phenomena grading imperceptibly into one another.

11. *Principle of Practicality:* A scientist expects that in any situation involving competition among units of varying potentialities, those which work best under existing circumstances will tend to survive and perpetuate themselves.

7

12. *Principle of Continuous Discovery:* A scientist hopes that it will be possible to go on learning more and more about the material world and the material universe of which it is a part, until eventually all may be understood.

13. *Principle of Complementarity:* A scientist attempts to incorporate all phenomena into a single, consistent, natural scheme, but he recognizes that contradictory generalizations may be necessary to describe different aspects of certain things as they appear to us.

14. *Principle of Social Limitation:* The social framework within which a scientist operates may determine and limit the kinds of problems on which he works, and the data which he collects, and may also influence his conclusions.

Step One: Formulate the Question

The first step in the scientific process is to identify the issues which are critical to your overall goal. What are the critical questions which need to be answered in order to solve the problem or relieve the concerns which are important to you? There are thousands of unanswered questions in your discipline. Many of them are not worth the time, effort, and money it would take to answer them; they are trivial questions. Some of them are unanswerable, at least in the immediate future, because they are too complex. If the question is so nebulous that you cannot even begin to guess at what the answer might be, it could be classified as an unanswerable question. Intuition plays a vital role in defining the question, especially if it is intuition based on experience. Insight comes to the prepared mind. Many scientists had seen mold on their Petri dishes, but it took the intuition of Sir Alexander Fleming's prepared mind to ask the critical questions which led to the discovery of penicillin.

Once a question has been formulated it often needs to be subdivided into a number of smaller, more manageable questions. Do the methods of stimulation and inhibition proposed by Margaret Rood really work? This is an interesting question, but it is too broad, too vague. Does two minutes of rapid brushing followed by thirty seconds of slow icing on the triceps of a spastic child with cerebral palsy placed in the inverted position facilitate motion in elbow extention as measured by active range of motion? This is the kind of question that you can begin to answer, and even that question must be narrowed down and provided with a definition of terms before it becomes a workable research question. The final question should be precise, grammatically correct, and should state exactly what you expect to learn as a result of the study.

8

Step Two: Review the Literature

The second step is to find out whether or not someone else has already answered your question convincingly; there is no point in reinventing the wheel. This step usually involves a systematic review of the literature to find out what other people have thought and done concerning your question. Before you accept the conclusion of other researchers, however, be sure to check the basis upon which they make their statements or conclusions. Is it their considered opinion, or is it a statement based upon the interpretation of data gathered in a scientific way? Are the authors' statements based on generalized experiences, or are they based on carefully controlled observation? The careful researcher should be able to distinguish these various types of conclusions in the literature. This systematic review of what is known generally takes place in the library. The library as a research tool is discussed in more detail in Chapter 10.

Step Three: Develop and Execute a Plan

The third step in the scientific method is to develop a plan for gathering reliable data from a set of controlled observations which answer the research question. This plan includes some form of measurement. The observations usually involve measuring some phenomena and recording the observations as numerical data. Much more will be said about the construction of this plan in Chapters 4 through 8. At this point it is important to realize that the researcher does not simply go out and gather facts; he makes and records observations according to a precise plan and in controlled ways which usually involve measurement.

Step Four: Interpret Your Data

After the research plan has been carried out, the data must be examined with an unbiased and critical eye. What do the data mean? What are their implications for your question? Data must be interpreted in light of the question you set out to answer. Is the answer one you had expected or is it different? What are all of the possible ways in which your research question could be answered on the basis of the data you have gathered? Of the possible conclusions, which one is most likely to be correct when all aspects of your experiment have been considered? What are your chances of being right if you answer your question in a certain way on the basis of your data? One uses every tool available in working with the data to arrive at their most probable meaning. Again, the intuition of the prepared mind is important. The light which the work of other people might shed on your data is important, and the rules of logic as tools for understanding are important. All of the ways of knowing contribute to the final interpretation and conclusion.

Step Five: Sharing Your Results

The final step in the validation of clinical practice is to share what you have learned with your colleagues. There are many ways of sharing: in-service educational programs in your department; state, regional, and national meetings of your professional association; newsletters and bulletins of the special interest groups within your profession; and professional journals. Crucial to all of these forms of sharing is the correct use of language. There are many good reference books on this: some of them are included in the bibliography at the end of the book. The ability to express your results is attained through practice, the same process that will refine your clinical skills.

PRACTICE

Turn now to Appendix C at the back of the book and read the article by Ayres. Read it fairly quickly this first time through; we will return to this article again and again as we progress through the textbook. See if you can identify the steps which are essential to a research project: the question, what other people have had to say about the question, the plan which guided the data collection, and the data interpretations made. Does the article fulfill the final step, i.e., is the report clearly written?

We will return to the second, third, and fourth steps in later chapters. Go back now and concentrate on the research question(s). See if you can define the question that this researcher was asking. (Hint: it is often expressed as the "purpose of the study.") Is the question clear to you from the way that it is reported in the article? If there are any unusual terms in the statement of the question, are they defined in the text so that you know precisely what the investigator means by them? What is the overall goal of this specific question being asked? What do you think the clinical significance of the question(s) might be? Do you think that an answer to the question would contribute to the basic knowledge of the profession and thus to the welfare of patients? Remember that most contributions will seem relatively insignificant. Nobel prize winners are few in number; highly significant breakthroughs in knowledge may occur only several times in a century, but these breakthroughs usually come because many people have answered many seemingly insignificant questions along the way which lead up to the big insight. Do not expect the author of the article to answer more than the question he has specified, but the reader should try to see how this bit of knowledge fits into the big picture.

You will find that the article by Ayres, like so many, will not clearly answer all the questions raised by this text. There are several reasons for this, some of which are practical. One important practical reason is the space limitation imposed on authors by editors. This limitation has become increasingly stringent in recent years with the rapidly rising costs of printing. The next time you are in the library stacks find a journal that has been in print for 60 years or so and compare an old article with a current one in terms of length and conciseness of expression; the limitations of the more recent article will be obvious.

Another reason for the missing answers is that most authors (and editors) assume that anyone interested enough in the topic to read the article will be familiar with standard terminology in the area of study. They also assume that their readers are sufficiently sophisticated in research methodology to understand some procedures implicitly. Both of these assumptions are often in error, and make research especially difficult for the neophyte of a discipline. For this reason you should have a good collegiate dictionary and a good medical dictionary at hand when you are studying the literature.

Since it is designed for students, this textbook will raise as many questions as possible. They will not all be applicable to every article. Their purpose is to alert you to possible areas of concern and points of interest as you learn to read professional literature. You will sometimes need to "read between the lines" to find answers. This is not necessarily a criticism of the article; it can be, rather, an instructive experience in logical thinking for you. On the other hand, some writers omit information for less noble reasons. Let us pass over them with the comment that in literature as in commerce, let the consumer beware.

ASSUMPTIONS

Every act which we perform rests on assumptions, which are accepted at face value without questioning. These assumptions underlie our behavior, yet we seldom give them a second thought. To give a simple example, I go barrelling down the highway at a speed of 55 miles/hour in the middle of the day on the assumption that the sun is going to continue to shine and that I will not, therefore, need to turn on the headlights. If this assumption should some day prove to be false, I might blindly run into a bridge or a tree. I perform this dangerous act daily without checking out several of the assumptions upon which it is based. In another example, I drive rapidly down the highway on the assumption that the car is going to continue to function in a safe manner. Many thousands of people have died when that assumption proved false; yet we cannot be expected to check out every assumption upon which we act.

As noted earlier in this chapter, the scientific method also makes some very important assumptions which are seldom checked out. They are "given" background for any scientific endeavor. There are, in addition, assumptions which are particular to each project. The careful researcher takes pains to identify the most important assumptions upon which each individual study is based. For example, if we were doing a study of the attitudes of hospitalized patients toward the therapy services in a hospital, one of the things that we would have to assume is that the patients answered honestly the questions which were put to them about the services. To be sure, the investigator should attempt to increase the probability that the patient will answer honestly. He might distribute an anonymous questionnaire—unsigned and unmarked—to be returned through the hospital mail system, the reasoning being that anonymity will increase the honesty of the responses. But since we cannot get inside the patient's head to examine his true feelings, after all precautions have been taken, we must assume that the patient has responded honestly since we cannot verify that he has.

It is important for the researcher to identify such assumptions; they contribute to the accuracy of his conclusions. It should be remembered, too, that whenever we deal with human subjects we encounter a multitude of variables which simply cannot be controlled. Assumptions can then be made about the regularity or distribution of those uncontrollable variables. This point will be dealt with more extensively in Chapter 3, in the section on sampling.

When we use electronic instruments we assume that after calibration they are functioning correctly and will record accurately. If we make a measurement on a patient two days in a row using the same machine, we assume the two measurements are comparable and that any changes which might be recorded are due to changes in the characteristic we are measuring and not to a change in the measuring device.

Carefully indentifying our assumptions often gives us clues to controls which we can apply to make our study more valid. For example, by identifying the assumption that an electronic instrument is functioning correctly, we are reminded to check the reliability of the instrument's calibration. Thus, the more assumptions we can identify in a given study, the more information we have to evaluate the results of that study.

In formal research reports, such as theses and dissertations, the assumptions underlying the study are usually stated quite clearly. However, in journal articles, where there is a premium on space, the assumptions are often unstated. In evaluating a report and making decisions about what actions you are going to take on the basis of the information contained therein, it is important to identify the unstated assumptions, and decide whether or not the assumptions are valid ones.

Return now to the article by Ayres. Are any assumptions identified in the text? Can you identify some of the unstated assumptions upon which the work was based? Based on what you know now, how would you evaluate these stated and unstated assumptions?

AUTHORITATIVE SOURCES

As stated earlier, it is important to review the available information which is relevant to your problem. But how is one to distinguish reliable from unreliable sources of information? An important distinction to be made here is that of primary versus secondary sources. If I say that I saw George hit Bill, I am a primary source of information about the incident. However, if I say that Betty told me that she saw George hit Bill, I am a secondary source of information; Betty would be the primary source. In terms of scientific literature, primary sources are those reports written by people who made the original observations upon which the conclusions were made. By and large, primary sources in the scientific community are the reports of original investigative studies. Secondary sources encompass the review of literature in a research article. The investigator reviews, in his report, what others have said that is relevant to his question. Another type of secondary source is a textbook, which organizes and summarizes primary sources, and interprets them according to the understanding of the textbook author.

Ideally, an investigator should never accept a secondary source if the primary sources are available. Secondary sources contain all of the possible errors, misinterpretations, or biases of the author of the primary source, as well as any misinterpretations or biases by the author of the secondary source. In addition, a secondary source may leave out essential information which will cause the reader to misinterpret what the original data and conclusions were. Secondary sources rarely give the original data from which conclusions were drawn, so that the reader is not able to judge the adequacy of the data for the conclusion or to evaluate the relevance of the data to the question.

Look again at the article by Ayres. Can you tell from reading her review of the relevant literature whether the authorities she quoted and the sources she used were primary or secondary? If you wanted to use this article as a foundation for your own study, what parts of this article would be primary information for you and what parts would be secondary? If you wanted to make important decisions based upon information supplied by this article as a secondary source, what could you do to strengthen the probability that you were making a good decision? If you use this article as a primary source for making a decision, what kinds of questions should you ask yourself about the information contained in this article before you decided to use it as the basis for a decision?

HYPOTHESES

More specific characteristics of hypotheses are treated in Chapters 5 through 8. At this time, let us identify only some of the more general characteristics. Blakiston's dictionary[4] defines hypothesis as a "supposition or conjecture put forth to account for known facts." In a general sense the hypothesis is the research question to be answered. However, many purists would insist that the word hypothesis applies only to experimental research. The approach in this text is that the research hypothesis is the question to be answered by the research project, regardless of which type of research is being undertaken (see Chapter 3 for definitions of research types).

In experimental research the hypothesis takes on two specialized forms which refine the question. One form is called the null hypothesis, the other is called the alternate or research hypothesis.

The alternate hypothesis in an experimental study should be expressible in the if/then form: If I do this to the patient, then the patient will respond in this way. In practice it usually takes the form of a declarative statement, i.e., active exercise increases measured range more than passive exercise does. Thus, the alternate hypothesis is an intelligent guess as to the nature of the answer to your basic question; it predicts the outcome of a certain treatment.

The null hypothesis is crucial to one specific step in the research procedure. The null hypothesis is called null because it makes a statement that there is no difference; it predicts that there will be no difference. The null hypothesis is important for only one reason; it is the only form of the question to which a statistical test can be applied. It can be understood as a question, is there a difference? If the answer is no, then the null hypothesis is supported and your alternate is rejected. If the answer to "Is there a difference" is yes, then you reject the null hypothesis and your alternate hypothesis is supported.

The following example illustrates the difference between the research and the null hypotheses.

Question: Will brief ice relieve spasticity to the point of increasing function?

Research Hypothesis (H_A): *If* an ice pack (20 °F) is placed to cover 90 percent of the body of spastic biceps brachi muscles in hemiplegic patients for 5 minutes, *then* active elbow extension will increase by at least 5 degrees with subject in a sitting position with the humerus abducted to 90 degrees.

Null Hypothesis (H_0): There will be *no difference* in active elbow extension between hemiplegic subjects that have had 5 minutes of ice pack applied to the biceps and those who have not received ice treatment. (Position, application, and temperature are assumed to be the same as in the research hypothesis.)

Now look at the article by Ayres. Can you identify null or alternate hypotheses? If one of these forms is missing, can you supply it?

Let's look at one more set of hypothetical examples. Let us suppose that two good friends, one a staff physical therapist and the other a staff occupational therapist in St. Hopeless Hospital, are interested in improving joint mobility in patients with physical disabilities. They decide to conduct a series of experiments with two purposes: (1) to evaluate the accuracy of various tools for measuring joint mobility, and (2) to evaluate several therapeutic procedures for increasing joint mobility. Out of these purposes they develop a series of research hypothesis or questions.

1. What measurement tools and what therapeutic methods are currently being used by therapists in hospitals and clinics across the country?

2. What is the reliability of "standard" manual goniometry as used by the therapists in St. Hopeless?

3. Do the medical records of St. Hopeless Hospital demonstrate the expected level of use of quantitative goniometry?

4. What is the most accurate measurement tool available for practical daily use?

5. Do goniometric measures of joint mobility predict the patient's level of functional ability?

6. Does heat applied prior to active exercise increase joint mobility more than active exercise alone?

7. Which is better for maintaining joint mobility in rheumatoid ar-

thritic patients: heat and active exercise twice daily, heat and passive and active exercises twice daily, or a functional activity program twice daily?

8. Does goniometric biofeedback training increase functional ability?

Can you convert questions 2, 5, 6, 7, and 8 into if/then statements? Here are 3 and 4 for examples.

3. If the medical records of St. Hopeless Hospital are accurate reflections of actual practice, and if the therapists recorded quantitative goniometric measurements at the intake and terminal patient visits, then those records demonstrate the minimal expected level of usage for patient evaluation.

4. If one instrument is more accurate than all others tested, then that accuracy will be demonstrated when tested against a known range.

For question 1 there is no null hypothesis. The null hypotheses for 2, 3 and 4 follow.

2. There will be no significant difference between two therapists at St. Hopeless in the independent measures of several joint ranges of motion using manual goniometers according to the techniques described by Hurt.[4]

3. There will be no significant difference between the expected and the actual usage of quantitative goniometry by occupational and physical therapists at St. Hopeless Hospital as demonstrated in the hospital's medical records.

4. There will be no significant difference between a known range and readings using any one of several goniometric tools, each of which is deemed practical for daily use.

Now try writing null hypotheses for questions 5, 6, 7, and 8. When we reconsider each of these questions in more detail in later chapters, we may polish and refine them considerably. That is how researchers normally work, identifying auxiliary problems, defining terms, and redefining hypotheses until they have a clear, answerable question.

REVIEW QUESTIONS

1. An intern says to you that he is surprised that people in your department are involved in research and asks you the purpose of research in your discipline and who should do it. How would you answer?

16

2. Define and illustrate four ways of "knowing." How does each contribute to the search for knowledge?
3. Define the following terms: research, concept, principle, data, statistics, and hypothesis. Give illustrations of each one from your professional discipline.
4. Differentiate between goal, purpose, and hypothesis.
5. Outline the scientific method. Using the article by Houser from Appendix C, illustrate the general method of scientific inquiry.
6. Look at the article by Houser in Appendix C. What is the purpose of this study? What are the research questions?
7. Look at the article by Houser in Appendix C. What assumptions are explicit? What assumptions are implicit?
8. Differentiate between primary and secondary sources. What are the major *potential* sources of error in primary sources? What are the major *potential* sources of error in secondary sources?
9. Look at the article by Houser. Identify the alternate hypothesis(es). Are the null hypotheses stated? What are the null hypotheses in this study?

REFERENCES

1. Pruden, E. L., et al.: Ins and outs of research: Problem to publication. Am. J. Med. Technol. 36:209, 1970.
2. Dickoff, J. W., and James, P. A.: Think Island. Unpublished paper presented at Physical Therapy Graduate Education Conference, 1972, Airlie, Virginia.
3. Hoerr, N. L., and Osol, A. (eds.): *Blakiston's New Gould Medical Dictionary*, ed. 2. McGraw-Hill, New York, 1956.
4. Hurt, S. P.: Joint measurement. Am. J. Occup. Ther. 1(4):209, 1(5):281, 2(1):13, 1948.

ADDITIONAL READING

Basmajian, J. V.: Professional survival: The role of research in physical therapy. Phys. Ther. 57:283, 1977.
Cerasoli, P. A., and Watkins, M. P.: Research and experience in an undergraduate physical therapy program. Phys. Ther. 57:24, 1977.
Conine, T. A.: Dilemmas of research in occupational therapy. Am. J. Occup. Ther. 26(2):81, 1972.
Crocker, L. M.: Linking research to practice: Suggestions for reading a research article. Am. J. Occup. Ther. 31(1):34, 1977.
Drew, L. J.: Introduction to Designing Research and Evaluation. Chapter 1. C. V. Mosby, St. Louis, 1976.
Edsall, F. et al.: A procedure for facilitating physical therapy research. Phys. Ther. 57:1138, 1977.
Erviti, V. F., and Scott, M.: Research design and statistics in an undergraduate physical therapy curriculum. Phys. Ther. 54:256, 1974.
Fowler, W. M.: Physical therapy and research. Phys. Ther. 49:977, 1969.
King, L. J.: Occupational therapy research in psychiatry: A perspective. Am. J. Occup. Ther. 32(1):15, 1978.
Lawrence, M.: Preparing for research in physical therapy. Phys. Ther. 46:42, 1966.

Leedy, P. D.: Practical Research: Planning and Design. Chapters 1 and 4. Macmillan, N.Y., 1974.

Lehmkuhl, D.: Let's reduce the understanding gap. Part I The question: what and why? Phys. Ther. 50:61, 1970.

Paolino, A. F.: Prospects for research in occupational therapy. Am. J. Occup. Ther. 16(4):167, 1962.

Reilly, M.: Research potentiality of occupational therapy. Am. J. Occup. Ther. 14(4): 206, 1960.

Worthingham, C. A.: Development of physical therapy as a profession through research and publication. Phys. Ther. 40:573, 1960.

Chapter 2

THE ROLE OF THEORY IN RESEARCH

OBJECTIVES

1. *Define theory, model, operational definition.*
2. *Discuss role of theory in research.*
3. *Discuss relationship between hypothesis, theory, and knowledge.*
4. *Define hypothetical construct.*
5. *Discuss essential components of a theory and illustrate them by outlining a limited or partial theory.*
6. *Define and illustrate taxonomy.*

THEORY

The central theme of this chapter is the concept of a theory. A *theory* is a set of principles (in this context often called postulates) which are based on solid evidence; a theory organizes what is known about the subject of the theory and it acts as a stimulus to research. Let us look at some of the essential characteristics of this definition of a theory.

First of all, it is a set of principles. You will recall from Chapter 1 that a principle is a statement of relationship between two or more concepts. If necessary it might serve the reader to go back to Chapter 1 and review the definitions of concepts and principles, for they are the building stones of a theory.

19

The next essential ingredient in our definition of a theory is that these principles are based on solid evidence. This evidence has often been reported in research studies and summarized in textbooks. This solid evidence is the body of facts possessed by a discipline or a profession, and it almost always includes the generally accepted interpretation of what those facts mean. Evidence is not hearsay; it is not opinion; it is the body of substantiated facts which are generally held to be true by respected professionals in a particular subject area.

The next critical ingredient in our definition of a theory is that it organizes what is known; here the word "organizes" places an emphasis on the relationships and interrelationships among the facts, concepts, and principles of a subject. A good theory should organize and encompass everything that is known about that particular subject. A good example of the organization of a theory is the Periodic Table of the Elements which people generally study in chemistry.

The Periodic Table organizes and summarizes the theory of chemical elements in tabular form, and graphically illustrates the relationships between the various elements (concepts) in the theory. Other examples of theory organization are the atomic theory of matter and the wave theory of light.

Most theories can be classified on at least two spectra. A theory may be anywhere along a spectrum which is at one end partial, specific, or limited and at the other is global and general. The same theory may also be classified as qualitative or quantitative; this latter classification is examined further in Chapter 4. An example of a large global theory is the germ theory of disease. The germ theory attempts to explain everything that is known about pathology in living organisms which is caused by other living organisms. However, it is not so global or all encompassing that it attempts to explain everything that is known about all disease and dysfunction; it is applicable only to those disorders caused by living organisms. So aneurysmatic strokes, for example, are not covered by the germ theory of disease.

The last element in our definition of a theory is that it acts as a stimulus to research which generates new principles. This element in the definition specifies the most important and most meaningful purpose of a theory. On the basis of the theory, predictive statements are made and then tested for accuracy. In the language of Chapter 1, we might say that *if* the theory is correct, *then* certain things will happen. The if/then statement becomes a hypothesis (which, within the context of theory, is often called a deduction). We can then set up an experiment which controls all factors except one; we observe that one factor or manipulate it or treat it in some way, and look to see if that manipulation or treatment produces the results that we predicted on the basis of the theory.

It cannot be emphasized too strongly that the major purpose of the theory is to stimulate the search for new facts, concepts, and principles which will either substantiate the theory or alter it in ways which will make it more accurate, more effective, more predictive, or more comprehensive. As noted earlier, one of the basic principles of this text is that research which grows out of theory is more likely to be useful and productive than is research which grows out of trial and error or happenstance. This is not to deny unexpected benefits of serendipity or the use of intuition, although fruitful intuition quite frequently comes to those who are well grounded in theory. Through the development of theory a hypothesis becomes substantiated to the point where it can be called a principle. In time the principle may be so widely accepted that it becomes a law.

Essential Components of a Theory

There are three essential components to a theory when it is formally stated. Table 2-1 is an example of a very limited theory; it explains a very specific and restricted set of phenomena. The three components shown are definitions, postulates, and deductions. You have already met all three of these under other names.

Definitions

Definitions are concepts, or become such when they are fully understood. Within a formal statement of a theory, a concept is defined very precisely—in language so concrete and technical that there is no question as to when and where it applies and when and where it does not apply. The definition should use terms which are so clear, concrete, and precise that one could divide everything in the world into those things that are included in the definition and those which are not, with no possible disagreement as to the inclusions or exclusions. A term often used for this kind of definition is *operational definition*. An operational definition refers to phenomena which are concrete, observable, and measurable at some level. The "at some level" will be dealt with more extensively in a later chapter.

Let us look at an example of an operational definition. A general dictionary definition of intelligence[1] is that it is the capacity to apprehend facts and propositions and their relations. That's fine as far as it goes, but how do you know it when you see it, and how do you measure it? It does not refer to concrete phenomena and therefore is not operationally defined. A much more concrete, specific, technical, and operational definition might be the followng. "For this study, intelligence is defined as the total score on the Stanford-Binet Test of Intelligence when administered in the standard, prescribed way." That definition points to a measurable score which can be recognized and compared. One can see how it would be possible to generate 10 or 15 different operational definitions of intelligence. Accordingly, when reading research materials it is often important to see what definition the author has used so that you will know whether or not it bears relevance to your area of interest. For example, if I were looking for articles on motor intelligence and I found a study which used the definition above, I probably would not pursue that article further. An important principle is contained here and it is well expressed by Travers: [11] ". . . one achieves more by being able to discuss limited phenomena with precision than by indulging in exchanges of vague generalities . . . ."

Postulates

The second essential element in a theory is a postulate (principle, generalization). Postulates state *demonstrated* relationships between the elements defined. In order to qualify as even a partial theory, a statement must have some principles based on valid, generally accepted evidence. Table 2-1 is deficient in this area, as stated in its footnote (*). Chapter 5 discusses what you can do if you have not reached the point where you can define even a limited theory in the area in which you are interested.

Deductions

The last essential element in the formal statement of a theory is the deduction, which, for research purposes, is our old friend, hypothesis. A deduction is a logical if/then inference derived from the principles. If proven, confirmed, and accepted by a significant proportion of the professional community it becomes a new postulate or principle. One deduction may eventually become a principle on its own, or it may be combined with a number of proven hypotheses to form a new principle.

Construction of adequate theory is a profoundly difficult but essential task ensuring that each research project grows out of the previous one in logical, developmental progression. To the degree that theory is effectively utilized, both human service practice and the process of research are facilitated.[12]

Table 2-1. Limited and partial theory of goniometry

Definitions*

1. Goniometry: art, process, or science of measuring angles.[1]
2. Goniometer: an instrument for measuring angles.[1]
3. Arthrometer: an instrument for measuring joints.[2]
4. Protractor arthrometer: two rigid shafts intersecting at a union allowing movement at right angles to their longitudinal axis; a protractor is fixed to one of these shafts so that its center corresponds with this union; the other shaft can move independently of the protractor and acts as an indicator.[2]
5. Diarthroidal articulation: a movable joint at the juncture of two or more bones.[3]
6. Axis of rotation: an imaginary line, itself at rest, about which a rotating limb turns in a plane at right angles to the axis.[4,5]
7. Joint center or fulcrum: the axis about which a bony lever pivots.[5,6]
8. Bony lever or limb segment: a rigid bar (bone) which pivots about a fixed point.[6]
9. Range of motion (ROM): quantitative measure of motion of bony levers at joint axes of rotation; measured in terms of that portion of an arc of motion which the moving limb segment describes on a hypothetical 360° circle.[7]
10. Active ROM: measurement of joint range achieved by active contraction of the governing muscles.[8]
11. Passive ROM: measurement of joint range achieved by the examiner when the governing muscles are relaxed.[8,9]
12. Normal ROM: a composite of normal ranges of joint mobility reported in the literature.[5,7-10]
13. Plane of motion: Sagittal, frontal, or transverse directions of movement from the anatomical position.[6,7]
14. Joint mobility: the ability to produce or allow a range of motion in diarthroidal articulations.

Postualtes**

1. An "ideal" method for determining ROM should allow the recording of accurate readings which are reproducible by different observers, and it should be applicable to all limb joints in people of different body dimensions.[2]
2. An adequate goniometer or arthrometer should be simple in construction and use, and should not interfere with joint movement.[2]
3. Compensatory motion at joints may interfere with accurate recordings, particularly at shoulder, forearm, back, hip, and ankle.[8]
4. Accurate measurement requires placing the union of the shafts of

the arthrometer over the axis of motion when the measurement is read.[5,8]

5. Accurate measurement requires placing the shafts of the arthrometer over or parallel to the bony lever and in the same plane of motion when the measurement is read.[5,8]

6. Goniometry is used to measure and record active and passive ranges of motion in patients with actual or potential loss of joint mobility.[2,8]

7. Goniometry is used in the evaluation of physical disability, in planning therapeutic interventions, and in evaluating therapy.[2,8]

8. It is often important to measure both the active and passive ranges of motion in a particular joint.[9]

9. All movements are measured from specified starting positions identical with the anatomical zero position except for radioulnar joints where midposition is zero.[5]

Deductions

1. If two therapists are trained in the same method of goniometry, then their recorded ROM on the same joints will be the same ±5 degrees (or their error is equal to or less than 5 degrees, or their separate measures will be correlated at a highly significant level).

2. If patients with reduced joint mobility demonstrate an increase in active ROM which is equal to or greater than 25 percent of their recorded loss, then they will concurrently demonstrate a significant increase in functional ability.

3. If a patient has a painful joint which demonstrates significantly less active than passive ROM, then 20 minutes of comfortable moist heat applied to the joint and its adjacent limb segments will significantly increase active ROM.

---

*These definitions are not fully exhaustive, for example, functional ability, physical disability, sagittal plane, frontal plane and transverse plane are concepts that are assumed rather than defined.

**"Postulates" 1 through 5 are based on reason and experience. Literature could not be found which produced experimentally based principles. This clearly weakens the "theory".

Properties of a Theory

Every theory has some generality in that it can be applied to more than one instance. Theories are about kinds or classes of phenomena rather than about unique or individual phenomena. A theory should be consistent in the sense that it does not contradict itself. And it should be complete; that is, its set of postulates should explain everything which the theory intends to explain, however global or limited that may be. A theory is useless if it is not testable, and it should be as simple as is commensurate with the task of being complete. This latter statement is sometimes called the law of parsimony.

No theory is ever final. It merely represents the current state of knowledge about a given topic. As more facts become available, more refined methods of experimentation and/or analysis and more refined observational techniques are developed; as more research is done, the theory changes and improves. New concepts relative to the topic may be incorporated into the definitions and new postulates and hypotheses formulated. Theory is not an affirmation; it is only a method of analysis. A theory may prove to be a formulation of one's ignorance, to be used as long as it is helpful and then discarded. Its function is to organize the available evidence in the search for better evidence.

One of the very useful functions of organizing and writing out what we know in theory form is that it helps us to see clearly what we really know, based on solid evidence (principles), and what we think we know (hypothesis). Dykes[13] has very forcefully called our attention to the problems created when we confuse hypothesis with knowledge (substantiated postulates). Dykes attributes much poor medical practice to this confusion; he says:

> Although there can be no scientific method without the hypothesis, a clear distinction must be made between a formulative, but untested hypothesis and a tested and accepted one. . . . Unfortunately, however, a report of a group of antedotal cases sometimes assumes the appearance of a bona fide structured, scientific investigation. . . . Thus, through lack of critical thinking, engendered by lack of time, material that should at best generate no more than a weak hypothesis, unfortunately may soon be offered as proof of a causal relationship.

Dykes recognizes that when pressed by the need to treat patients, one must often proceed on hypotheses that are untested or poorly supported. However, if one recognizes clearly the status of the hypothesis on which one treats the patient, then the way is laid for the scientific testing and eventual validation or rejection of that hypothesis. In addition to the article by Kielhofner in Appendix C, other theory articles in the literature include Harris and Adams (see list of additional reading at the end of this chapter) although Adams is probably not for the beginning reader of theory.

25

MODEL

Sometimes a theory may grow out of a more speculative working model. A *model* represents complex phenomena in a simpler way. Examples are the globe as a model of the earth, a road map, a table of organization for a hospital, or an architect's plans for a building; these are replica models. Sometimes a model is expressed as an analogy, for example, a molecule is like the universe. Sometimes hypothetical constructs become models; these are symbolic models.

A *hypothetical construct* is a verbal symbol for something which cannot be seen. Examples are intelligence, motivation, facilitation, inhibition, mechanical ability, physical therapy, occupational therapy, etc. None of these things can be seen. We infer their existence as causes behind specific behaviors which we observe. It is possible to see an occupational therapist, and it is possible to see a patient who is receiving something called occupational therapy, but you can ot see occupational therapy per se. Its existence is inferred from wha we see and therefore it is called a hypothetical construct. It is a con pt constructed from a hypothesis regarding the causation of things seen. Occupational therapy is a symbolic model for a group of related behaviors.

Figure 2-1 is a model of empirical knowledge, which is a hypothetical construct. You can't see, taste, touch, or directly measure knowledge. It is inferred from what *people* say and do. It is measured indirectly through tests of what a *person* or many people say, write, or do. But knowledge itself is a hypothetical construct. Figure 2-1 describes both content and process. If it is an adequate model, all em-

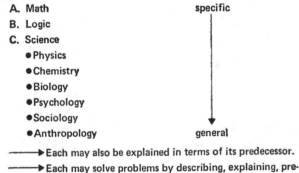

A. Math   specific
B. Logic
C. Science
   ● Physics
   ● Chemistry
   ● Biology
   ● Psychology
   ● Sociology
   ● Anthropology   general

——▶ Each may also be explained in terms of its predecessor.
——▶ Each may solve problems by describing, explaining, predicting, controlling.

D. Philosophy

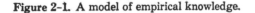

Figure 2-1. A model of empirical knowledge.

pirical knowledge can be classified according to the model and no empirical knowledge will be left out. This model could be used to develop a theory of empirical knowledge, which would be more useful for generating new knowledge. The interested student may find other models in the literature, for example, Heard and Payton (see "Additional Reading").

TAXONOMY

The word taxonomy is derived from two Greek words which translate as "the law of arrangement." One of the earliest and certainly the most famous taxonomy was that of Linnaeus, and the word, taxonomy, has been so identified with the Linnaean taxonomy that *Blakistons Medical Dictionary*[3] defines taxonomy as "the science of the classification of organisms." However, the word has a more generic meaning as the science of classification of any set of related phenomena. In education there are two very famous taxonomys, *Bloom's Taxonomy of Educational Objectives in the Cognitive Domain*[14] and *Krathwohl's Taxonomy of Educational Objectives in the Affective Domain.*[15] A much lesser known companion to these two is *Harrow's Taxonomy of the Psychomotor Domain.*[16] One of the major advantages of a taxonomy is that it gives one a quick overview of an entire field of study or area of interest in a way which elucidates the relationships between components of that field. For example, one can find a chart of the animal kingdom based on the Linnaean taxonomy which summarizes on one large page all of the animals known to man and how they are related to one another with regard to key anatomical and/or physiological characteristics. In a sense, a taxonomy is a special form of a model; like the Table of Elements, a taxonomy can provide the astute observer with clues which may lead to the discovery of important information. In Chapter 11 we will pursue theory further in reference to the therapeutic disciplines.

REVIEW QUESTIONS

1   What is a theory and what are the essential components of a theory?
2. How does theory aid research?
3. What is a model; how does it relate to theory?
4. What is a hypothetical construct; how does it relate to theory?
5. What is a taxonomy; how does it relate to theory?
6. Look at the article by Kielhofner in Appendix C.
    a. Define the key critical concept of the article.

27

b. Find and/or define other concepts necessary for a theory of temporal adaptation.
c. List the postulates (principles) supported by some evidence, as presented in the article.
d. Write several alternate hypotheses based on the definitions and postulates. Use the two case histories presented in the article to help form hypotheses.

REFERENCES

1. Webster's Seventh New Collegiate Dictionary. G & C Merriam Co., Springfield, 1963.
2. Salter, N.: Methods of measurement of muscle and joint function. J. Bone Joint Surg. 378:3:474, 1955.
3. Hoerr, N. L., and Osol, A. (eds.): Blakiston's New Gould Medical Dictionary. McGraw Hill, N.Y., 1956.
4. Dyson, G.: The Mechanics of Athletics, ed. 4. University of London Press, 1967.
5. Moore, M. L.: The measurement of joint motion. Part II: The technique of goniometry. Phys. Ther. 29:256, 1949.
6. Kelley, D. L.: Kinesiology: Fundamentals of Motion Description. Prentice-Hall, Englewood Cliffs, N.J., 1971.
7. Poland, J. L., Hobard, D. J., and Payton, O.D.: The Musculoskeletal System. Medical Examination Publishing Co., Flushing, N.Y., 1977.
8. Hurt, S. P.: Joint measurement. Am. J. Occup. Ther. 1:4:209, 1947; 1:5:281, 1947; and 2:1:13, 1948.
9. American Orthopaedic Association: Manual of Orthopaedic Surgery. Chicago, 1972.
10. American Academy of Orthopaedic Surgeons: Measuring and Recording Joint Motion. Chicago, 1965.
11. Travers, R. M. W.: An Introduction to Educational Research, ed. 3. Macmillan Co. London, 1969.
12. Twain, D.: "Developing and implementing a research strategy." In Struening, E. L. and Guttentag, M. (eds.): Handbook of Evaluation Research. Sage Publications, Beverly Hills, CA, 1975, pp. 27-52.
13. Dykes, M. H. M.: Uncritical thinking in medicine: The confusion between hypothesis and knowledge. *JAMA* 227(11): 1275, 1974.
14. Bloom, B. J., et al. (eds.): Taxonomy of Educational Objectives. Handbook I: Cognitive Domain. David McKay Co., N.Y., 1956.
15. Krathwohl, D. R., et al.: Taxonomy of Educational Objectives. Handbook II: Affective Domain. David McKay Co., N.Y., 1964.
16. Harrow, A. J.: A Taxonomy of the Psychomotor Domain. David McKay Co., N.Y., 1972.

ADDITIONAL READING

Adams, J. A.: A closed—loop theory of motor learning. *J. Motor Behav.* 3:2:111, 1971.
Harris, F. A.: Inapproprioception: A possible sensory basis for athetoid movements. Phys. Ther. 51:761, 1971.
Heard, C.: Occupational role acquisition: a perspective on the chronically disabled. Am. J. Occup. Ther. 31(4):243, 1977.
Mosey, A. C.: An alternative: The biopsychosocial model. Am. J. Occup. Ther. 28(3):137, 1974.
Payton, O. D., et al.: Quality of patient care and a peer review system: a model. Phys. Ther. 51:296, 1971.

Stein, F.: Three facets of psychiatric occupational therapy: models for research. Am. J. Occup. Ther. 23(6):491, 1969.

Travers, R. M. W.: An Introduction to Educational Research, ed. 3. Chapters 1 and 2. Macmillan, London, 1969.

Chapter 3

INTRODUCTION TO RESEARCH DESIGN

OBJECTIVES

1. *Define research design, population, sample, and treatment groups.*
2. *Define and discuss the general concepts of control and sampling.*
3. *List the essential characteristics of descriptive research, correlational research, and predictive research.*
4. *Distinguish between basic and applied research.*

RESEARCH DESIGN

You will recall that in Chapter 1 research was defined as a process for finding specific answers to specific questions in an organized, objective, and reliable way. Research *design* refers to those concepts and techniques which make research organized, objective, and reliable. Research design may be perceived as the mechanics by which the project is organized. In this context *organized* means that the relationships between the various components of the project are stated clearly; *objective* and *reliable* mean stating what you did so clearly and in such concrete terms that you or other people could repeat the same study and get the same results. Therefore, the two key elements in research design are: defining terms and defining relationships. These defini-

31

tions must be in operational terms as discussed in Chapter 2. Several common designs will be discussed in Chapters 5 through 8.

CONTROL

One of the most important concepts in research design is control. Control is particularly crucial to predictive research, but also has a part to play in correlational and descriptive research. The basic principle is that you should attempt to control *all* aspects of the research project *except* the one you are studying. For example, if you have designed a project to compare treatment A with treatment B, you will collect data on the effects of the two treatments and expect to interpret your data in such a way that you can answer the question: Which is better, treatment A or treatment B? You will not be able to make this clear-cut interpretation unless you have controlled your observations; i.e., your data collection, so that differences in the data can only be attributed to one of the two treatments and not to some other influence which you have failed to eliminate or control.

Go back to the example in Chapter 1 where we were looking at the effects on active elbow extension of 5 minutes of ice pack applied to the spastic biceps of a hemiplegic patient. Here, treatment A was the ice pack and treatment B was no treatment. Suppose that you collected data from a group of hemiplegic patients using this design and it appeared from looking at your data that the patients who received the ice did, indeed, extend their elbows actively to a greater extent than did the patients who did not receive the ice. Can you conclude from the data that 5 minutes of ice pack inhibits spasticity and thus facilitates active excursion by the antagonistic muscle? Suppose on closer investigation you discover that most of the patients who got the ice pack had a mild spasticity with good active contraction of the triceps whereas most of the patients who received no treatment were severe spastics with only trace active motion in their triceps. Would you still be able to interpret your data in the same way? Obviously in such a study one of the controls should demonstrate approximately the same degree of spasticity in both groups. Suppose one group was composed primarily of young alert, traumatic hemiplegics, while the other group was composed primarily of old, senile hemiplegics who had suffered cardiovascular accidents; would not that influence your interpretation?

The two examples given above should help to clarify the point that in a good research study as many variables as possible are controlled, except the variables under study—in the case discussed here, icing—so that any differences which result from the treatment can be attributed to that treatment and not to some uncontrolled variable operating on the subjects.

In health sciences research a number of variables which are frequently important come readily to mind: age, sex, severity and length of time since onset of illness, type and dosages of medications, psychological and socioeconomic factors, in-patient or out-patient status, the presence or absence of other diseases or disabilities, and numerous other factors revealed in a good history and physical examination. However, effective control can never be applied in a routine and mechanical way. Each research project, each question, and each research design needs to be evaluated carefully to define exactly what variables are to be studied and what other variables must be controlled so that they do not contaminate the data or distort the interpretation.

This emphasis on control appears again and again throughout this text as we discuss specific research designs and also when we discuss the threats to internal and external validity in Chapter 9. Look at paragraph 4 in Houser and Johnson's article (Appendix C). Three controls are stated clearly: all of the subjects in the sample were boys; they were all wheelchair-bound, and they all had a diagnosis of pseudohypertrophic muscular dystrophy. Two other less specific controls are contained in the same paragraph: the subjects ranged in age from 8 to 15—this clearly eliminated young children and all adults—and they were all referred to physical therapy while attending a school for handicapped children. Presumably, the school had some criteria for admission which further homogenized the sample, and the fact that they all needed physical therapy (and, by inference, pulmonary physical therapy as well) tells us that they all had a pathosis in need of that particular kind of therapeutic intervention.

In paragraph 7 Houser defines additional controls which were placed on her sample. Individuals were matched on the basis of one of the pulmonary function tests and then the members of each matched pair were randomly divided into two groups. In the last half of paragraph 7 Houser provides averages which reflect the outcome of her attempt to normalize the variables of vital capacity and age. Paragraph 8 and Table 2 outline other controls which helped to equate the two groups. Paragraph 9 makes it clear that both groups received exactly the same treatment except for the variables under study. The variables under study are described in paragraphs 10 through 14. Can you find descriptions of similar controls in the Ayres study?

SAMPLING

A second concept which is crucial to all research designs is the concept of sampling. A *population* refers to the members of a well-defined class of people, events, or objects which are the focus of an investigation.[1] A *sample* is composed of those subjects selected from a population for research study. To collect data on a group of people, objects, or events and be interested in the interpretation of the data only as it applies to those individuals who were studied is unusual. Almost always, one hopes that the interpretation can be extrapolated to the larger group of people or events from which the sample was taken. In order to make this inference from the sample to the population, it is important that the sample be appropriate to the research question and representative of the population.

Defining the appropriate population for a given study is not always as easy as it may seem. For example, the therapists at St. Hopeless Hospital may decide to do a study and draw their sample from those hemiplegic patients who were admitted as in-patients to the hospital during a calendar year, and their final report may interpret the results as if the population were all hemiplegic patients in the world. But is that really so? *Theoretically,* each individual in the population should have an equal opportunity to be in the sample drawn for study. But in this hypothetical example even the hemiplegic patients admitted to the hospital across the street did not have the opportunity to be in the study, let alone hemiplegics across the country or halfway around the world. Therefore, an accurate definition of the population of this study is the hemiplegic patients admitted to St. Hopeless Hospital. We need not be so rigid as to further define the population as those patients admitted during a specified calendar year; however, on the other extreme, we might also not want to include in the population all hemiplegic patients admitted to St. Hopeless if it were founded in 1892; too many factors, both medical and sociological, would have changed over such a long period of time. The population should be similar to the sample in all respects except the one under study, in this case, the independent variable would be the application of therapeutic procedures selected for study.

The example in the paragraph above illustrates some of the difficulties involved in defining the population of the study. Some researchers are more restrictive than others in this regard; since in most things virtue stands between the two extremes, the approach of this text will be that the population is that group of objects, individuals, or events which resemble the sample in all or the most important characteristics. Defining those important characteristics is the major difficulty when selecting a sample. Nevertheless, one should never abandon common sense while doing research. If St. Hopeless were a hospital serving primarily middle-class white Americans, and if it had

34

been designated "first class" by the American Hospital Association, then it might be logical to define the population to which the results of the study could be extrapolated as all white middle-class patients who were admitted to first-class hospitals in the United States in the late 1970s. As the details of the study develop, other limitations on population description may emerge.

One could also do a study in which the sample of five people was identical to the total population of five people, the five people being staff therapists in a given department. It could be a descriptive study to answer the question "How do they spend their time?" The behavior observed could be everything performed on the job during one week's time. It could be recorded through a task description by a trained observer. The results could prove very beneficial to patient care by suggesting better utilization of the therapists' time. The results might not be applicable to a hospital across the street which may have a totally different approach to organization and management. Thus, the characteristics of the sample and the population from which it is taken are crucial. The researcher must first identify his goals and purposes; then define the question and polish a hypothesis. He can then address himself to the questions of what population is appropriate and how a sample can be correctly chosen from that population.

The population and the sample must have the same scope and limitations. Many authors specifically state a number of characteristics which exclude many subjects from their study. If characteristics such as mental retardation and cerebral palsy were excluded from the sample, then obviously they would be excluded from the population to which the conclusions may be extrapolated. If the question concerns the motor development of children during the first year of life after premature birth, then obviously neither population nor sample would include two-year-olds or infants who were delivered after a normal-term pregnancy. Mistakes in this area are perhaps more frequently made by readers than by writers. As you learn to read scientific literature, it is wise to keep this issue in mind so that you do not extrapolate the findings of the study to a population beyond that intended by the author, or, more importantly, beyond that justified by the sample and the data collected.

Idealized Sampling Procedures

In this section the theoretical and mathematical ideals governing the concept of sampling are described. A later section deals with the application of these models to clinical research.

Theoretically, every individual in a population is identified and listed. This list is sometimes called a frame. For example, if the population under study were every registered republican in the state of Virginia, it should be possible to make a frame listing the names and addresses of every single person in the population. Since this number would be in the thousands it might be logistically and economically impractical to examine each individual in that population. Therefore, the researcher could decide to choose a sample of 300 from the described population.

In the theory of sampling it is important that each and every member of the population have an equal opportunity to be in the sample. There are several ways to draw such a sample. The simplest and most direct is to put each person's name (or an identifying number) on a slip of paper, thoroughly jumble up all of the names and then randomly draw from the box until 300 names are drawn. The purist would also shake the box up between each of the 300 draws.

Figure 3–1 is taken from a table of random numbers. To use this table you close your eyes and put your finger anywhere on the table. The number your have located in this way is your beginning point; you than proceed down the list taking every number between 1 and 45,000 until you have selected 300. You would then have randomly selected a sample of 300 (n) from your population of 45,000 (N).

Another method of obtaining a sample would be to randomly choose 30 counties out of the state and then randomly choose 10 subjects out of the registered republicans in each of the 30 counties in order to reach the desired n for your sample. Some people would contend that in this procedure the population had been redefined as those registered republicans in the 30 selected counties. However, if both the 30 counties and the 100 representatives were selected in random fashion, there is little reason to believe that the redefined population is not also representative of the theoretically larger population of the whole state.

Since our defined population is registered republicans in the state, and our sample has been chosen from registered republicans in the state, we have clearly met the criterion for appropriate subjects, but are they representative? The most powerful tool for assuring representativeness is that of randomization which is based on the law of chance. If the sample is randomly chosen from the population, then the law of chance dictates that the sample is almost always representative of the population. However, since "almost always" is not an absolute guarantee it is wise to double-check whenever possible.

Stratified Random Sampling

Going back to the method using 10 subjects from each of 30 counties, suppose that just by chance none of the 30 counties chosen in-

Random Numbers

1368	9621	9151	2066	1208	2664	9822	6599	6911	5112
5953	5936	2541	4011	0408	3593	3679	1378	5936	2651
7226	9466	9553	7671	8599	2119	5337	5953	6355	6889
8883	3454	6773	8207	5576	6386	7487	0190	0867	1298
7022	5281	1168	4099	8069	8721	8353	9952	8006	9045
4576	1853	7884	2451	3488	1286	4842	7719	5795	3953
8715	1416	7028	4616	3470	9938	5703	0196	3465	0034
4011	0408	2224	7626	0643	1149	8834	6429	8691	0143
1400	3694	4482	3608	1238	8221	5129	6105	5314	8385
6370	1884	0820	4854	9161	6509	7123	4070	6759	6113
4522	5749	8084	3932	7678	3549	0051	6761	6952	7041
7195	6234	6426	7148	9945	0358	3242	0519	6550	1327
0054	0810	2937	2040	2299	4198	0846	3937	3986	1019
5166	5433	0381	9686	5670	5129	2103	1125	3404	8785
1247	3793	7415	7819	1783	0506	4878	7673	9840	6629
8529	7842	7203	1844	8619	7404	4215	9969	6948	5643
8973	3440	4366	9242	2151	0244	0922	5887	4883	1177
9307	2959	5904	9012	4951	3695	4529	7197	7179	3239
2923	4276	9467	9868	2257	1925	3382	7244	1781	8037
6372	2808	1238	8098	5509	4617	4099	6705	2386	2830
6922	1807	4900	5306	0411	1828	8634	2331	7247	3230
9862	8336	6453	0545	6127	2741	5967	8447	3017	5709
3371	1530	5104	3076	5506	3101	4143	5845	2095	6127
6712	9402	9588	7019	9248	9192	4223	6555	7947	2474
3071	8782	7157	5941	8830	8563	2252	8109	5880	9912
4022	9734	7852	9096	0051	7387	7056	9331	1317	7833
9682	8892	3577	0326	5306	0050	8517	4376	0788	5443
6705	2175	9904	3743	1902	5393	3032	8432	0612	7972
1872	8292	2366	8603	4288	6809	4357	1072	6822	5611
2559	7534	2281	7351	2064	0611	9613	2000	0327	6145
4399	3751	9783	5399	5175	8894	0296	9483	0400	2272
6074	8827	2195	2532	7680	4288	6807	3101	6850	6410
5155	7186	4722	6721	0838	3632	5355	9369	2006	7681
3193	2800	6184	7891	9838	6123	9397	4019	8389	9508
8610	1880	7423	3384	4625	6653	2900	6290	9286	2396
4778	8818	2992	6300	4239	9595	4384	0611	7687	2088
3987	1619	4164	2542	4042	7799	9084	0278	8422	4330
2977	0248	2793	3351	4922	8878	5703	7421	2054	4391
1312	2919	8220	7285	5902	7882	1403	5354	9913	7109
3890	7193	7799	9190	3275	7840	1872	6232	5295	3148
0793	3468	8762	2492	5854	8430	8472	2264	9279	2128
2139	4552	3444	6462	2524	8601	3372	1848	1472	9667
8277	9153	2880	9053	6880	4284	5044	8931	0861	1517
2236	4778	6639	0862	9509	2141	0208	1450	1222	5281
8837	7686	1771	3374	2894	7314	6856	0440	3766	6047
6605	6380	4599	3333	0713	8401	7146	8940	2629	2006
8399	8175	3525	1646	4019	8390	4344	8975	4489	3423
8053	3046	9102	4515	2944	9763	3003	3408	1199	2791
9837	9378	3237	7016	7593	5958	0068	3114	0456	6840
2557	6395	9496	1884	0612	8102	4402	5498	0422	3335

Figure 3-1. Part of a table of random numbers. Reprinted with permission from: Owen, D. B.: Handbook of Statistical Tables. Addison-Wesley, Reading, Mass., 1962.

cluded any of the large cities in the state. The sample has then been biased in favor of the rural areas. A technique for correcting this error is called *stratified random sampling*. For example, if you have reason to believe that dwellers in the large city complexes are different in some of the important parameters that you wish to measure from those who dwell in rural areas, then you would take steps to make sure that both subgroups, urban and rural, are represented in your sample. One approach would be to identify all republicans in the state as either city dwellers or urban dwellers and then draw an equal number individuals from each group. Or, if you know from other sources that 40 percent of the state's population dwells in major cities and 60 percent in rural areas and small towns, you could draw a proportional stratified sample: 120 people from the urban list (40 percent of 300) and 180 (the other 60 percent) from the rural list.

Stratification can be used as long as the number of individuals in each stratified sample does not drop too low. For example, you might want to further stratify both the urban and rural populations into males and females, if you had a good reason to believe that this was an important differentiation for your study. The guiding principle is that the method of sampling chosen must be the one which offers the best possibility of giving you a sample which is truly representative of the general population (Fig. 3-2).

Systematic Sampling

Yet another option is known as *systematic sampling*. If you had a list of all 45,000 registered republicans in the state of Virginia and you wanted a sample of five percent (2250), you could enter a table of ran-

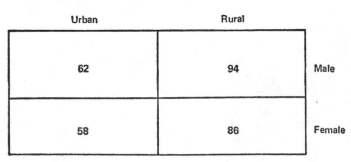

N=45,000 Registered Republicans in Virginia
n=300 Sample

	Urban	Rural	
	62	94	Male
	58	86	Female

Figure 3-2. Number of individuals in each of four classifications (cells) based on a two-way stratification of a sample.

dom numbers, (Fig. 3-1) until you located a number from 1 to 20. If this procedure gives you a number of 13, then you would begin with the 13th person on the list of the population as your first subject. You would then take every 20th person on the list.

Cluster Sampling

Another procedure is called *cluster sampling*. Using this technique you would select (by either drawing out of a hat or using a table of random numbers) every tenth county in the state. You would then use all of the registered republicans in that county as a part of your sample. This procedure is sometimes used when the population is composed of students and they are collected in clusters in schools. For example, you might randomly select 10 of the physical or occupational therapy schools in the United States, and then test all of the students in the schools thus selected. (Or all of the junior students, or all of the senior female students, or all of the faculty, etc.)

Double Sampling

The last form of sampling to be illustrated is *double sampling*. To continue with our hypothetical sample of registered republicans in the state of Virginia, you might send a questionnaire to the 300 selected individuals and ask them 10 preliminary questions. One of these might be "Did you vote in the last general election?" Let us say, for the sake of illustration, that 122 of the respondents indicated that they did vote in the last general election. You could then send these 122 people a longer and more detailed questionnaire, pursuing the issues pertinent to the objectives of your study. This is an example of double sampling. It is most useful in descriptive survey types of research. Some of the problems and limitations of survey samples are discussed in Chapter 5.

As noted earlier, randomization is the most powerful tool we have for imposing control on the process of sampling. Wherever possible randomization should be used not only to obtain a sample from a population, but also to divide the sample into different groups or to assign different treatments. If two or more groups are to be formed from the sample, the purpose of random assignment of subjects to different conditions or treatment groups is to form groups which are equivalent to each other in as many pre-experimental conditions as possible. Only then can differences be attributed to the treatment procedures. In both instances, sampling and group assignment, the process of chance is fundamental.

It should be noted here that chance in research does not imply haphazardness. Chance is used in research as part of a carefully planned and carefully executed technique, just as the table of random numbers has been carefully compiled.

Sequential Assignment

If samples cannot be chosen and group assignments made all at once as indicated in the ideal sampling procedures noted above, then the experimenter must assign individuals in a sequential fashion over a period of time rather than at the beginning of the experiment. In sequential assignment to groups, a modification of the hat technique can be used. If, for example, you are forming three treatment groups and you want n equal to 30 (10 people from each group), then you can write the number 1 (for treatment group 1) on 10 pieces of paper, the number 2 (for group 2) on 10 pieces of paper, and the number 3 (for group 3) on 10 pieces of paper, shuffle them thoroughly in the hat and draw them out, writing the numbers down one at a time as they are drawn. Say the resulting sequence begins: 3, 1, 1, 3, 2, 1. Then the first person to enter your experiment would go in group three, the second and third persons would go into group one, the fourth person to group three, and so on. You can also enter a table of random numbers and record in sequence each time you come upon a one, two, or three, and then assign subjects according to that sequence.

Once your experimental and control groups have been formed you should check to make sure that your randomization has produced homogenous groups. There are statistical methods for doing this, and occasionally you will see these "tests of homogeneity" reported in articles attesting to the fact that the groups observed were reasonably similar to each other.

Assignment by Matching

Sometimes it is not possible to control a sample through randomization. An alternate procedure is called *matching*. With this technique the researcher imposes his own criteria and attempts to force the groups into equivalency along dimensions or characteristics which the researcher believes to be important.

The first step in this approach is to identify the important characteristics. Let us say that age is considered by you, the researcher, to be a crucial factor for two groups of subjects. Using matching, you can impose this restriction on groups or individuals.

If you match groups, then you want both groups to have the same average (mean) age and the same age variations (a statistical measure of variation called variance is defined in Chapter 5). The concern here is that the mean ages and variances of the two groups are equal. This technique might be used to equate a senior physical therapy class and a senior occupational therapy class. Individuals may sometimes be moved from one group to another in order to insure this balance in age in a study which compared, for example, two halves of a senior class in school.

If you match individual pairs, you find two individuals who are very similar to each other with regard to crucial variables which you want to control. You than randomly assign each individual to one of the two groups. Let us say, again, that age is an important factor in the criteria which identify your sample. When you find two 31-year-old people who meet the criteria for admission into your sample, you randomly assign one to the first group and the other to the second group. You then may find two people 24 years old and randomly assign one to each group, and so on.

Notice that matching on critical variables is used for control, as a substitute for the control of chance. Chance still plays a minor part in selecting which of each pair would go to each group. If you have three or more groups, you must find three or more individuals who are alike with regard to the crucial variable which you want to control. You may also match on more than one controlling variable; for example, you might match two 30-year-old white females.

In both group and individual matching procedures it is important to have strong evidence of an important relationship between the matched variable and the experimental task.

A major limitation of this process is that once you get beyond two variables it becomes extremely difficult to find matching pairs; if you are matching triplets it is even more difficult. On a practical level, then, one is often limited to two groups matched on one or two critical variables, and therein lie the major flaws of this technique. First of all, it is difficult to identify all of the critical variables which you need to control. Secondly, there is a possibility that by matching individuals you introduce a systemic bias. Especially when you are working with human beings whose characteristics are so complex, it is practically impossible to control all relevant factors except through randomization. For these reasons many researchers say that matching should never be used as a substitute for randomization, and most would agree that you should never use matching if randomization is possible.

Individuals are sometimes matched during the course of an experimental task which involves repeated measures. Let us say that you plan to take three measures of shoulder range of motion; in the beginning, in the middle, and at the end of your experimental treatment. It might be possible to match individuals on the actual performance level

41

of the task itself so that a person with 100 degrees of active flexion of the shoulder would be matched with another person with 100 degrees of active flexion of the shoulder; these two would then be randomly assigned to two treatment protocols. In like manner two patients with only 15 degrees of active flexion would be randomly assigned to the same two treatment groups. *All other factors being equal*, it would then be reasonable to assume that differences between the individuals of a pair in your second and third measures of range of motion could be attributed to treatment technique, since they both started out at the same level. However, with this procedure we also run into the problem of compounding variables such as length of time the tightness has existed in the shoulder, severity of the disease process, motivation, and other factors which may tend to destroy the equality between a pair. Thus, matching should be avoided whenever other sampling methods are possible.

In the article by Houser (Appendix C) paragraphs 7 and 8 contain the methods by which she matched pairs in her study. Note that once the matching had been done the sample was divided into experimental and control groups using a table of random numbers. At the end of paragraph 7 and in Tables 1 and 2 she indicates the extent to which the *groups* (Table 2) and the individual *pairs* (Table 1) are homogenous. For example, in Table 1 the important characteristics of the individuals in pair 1 are given: age, functional groupings, and forced vital capacity. How did Ayres select her sample, and from what population? How do you think she used randomization? Into how many groups was Ayres' sample divided?

Figure 3-3 illustrates some of the basic ideas of research design which we have discussed. A population is identified as carefully as possible. It is all the people, objects, or events to which the results of a study might be relevant. From that population a sample is drawn. Ideally, complete *randomization*, which utilizes the laws of chance, will produce a truly representative sample of the population. As a researcher you are going to "do something" with or to that sample. You may treat the entire sample as one group or you may divide it (hopefully by randomization) into several treatment groups. The treatment may consist merely of observation in a natural setting (this would be your control group) or it may require experimental manipulation and observation.

The question of how many groups constitute the sample is an important issue in later chapters which deal more specifically with research design. It is important to realize that the criterion measures discussed in Chapter 4 may be taken once, twice or many times on each group. Unfortunately, the taking of criterion measures is sometimes called

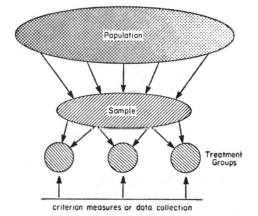

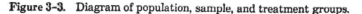

criterion measures or data collection

Figure 3-3. Diagram of population, sample, and treatment groups.

data sampling, and is not to be confused with the topic of this chapter, population sampling. Three data collections, one from each of three treatment groups within a sample, are illustrated in Figure 3-3.

SAMPLE SIZE

One of the most common questions asked by beginning researchers is "How large a sample do I need?" There is no clear-cut answer to that question. A rule of thumb which doesn't offer much help is that the larger the sample, the better. A more helpful rule is that the greater the variation in the population (and therefore in a representative sample), the larger the number needed in the sample.

The requirements of the statistical tools must also be considered in the question of sample size. Some statistical tests require a minimum number in each group. Statistical formulas can help to determine the appropriate sample size for a given set of criteria. Whenever possible, it is wise to consult someone familiar with these methods.

TYPES OF RESEARCH

No classification of research types is universally accepted. In this text we will divide all research into three major types: descriptive, correlational, and predictive (experimental). Chapters 4 through 6 discuss these types individually and identify their various subdivisions. For now, a quick overview of their similarities and differences will suffice.

First, let us look at the similarities. All three involve a question to be answered, but the questions themselves are different. All three have a

43

population, and all three look at a sample taken from the population (or in cases of very small populations, the sample may be the total population). All three collect data from the sample; they differ in the kinds of data they collect and the way they go about collecting them. Finally, all three interpret their data in an attempt to find the most likely and reasonable answer to the question. As Leedy[2] has so clearly pointed out, no amount of data collection, fact-finding, or fact-transcribing "can be dignified by the term research. . . . The mind of the researcher must do battle with the observed fact . . . until the fact reveals its inner significance," that is, its relation to the question being asked. So all types of research ask a specific question, search for the answer in an organized and planned way, and answer the question through interpretation of the data collected.

How do these three basic types of research differ? *In general* they differ (1) in the kind of question asked, (2) in the degree to which the sample is manipulated by the experimenter, (3) in the statistical tools used to summarize and/or interpret the data, and (4) in the formal properties of the predictions made on the basis of the data.

For descriptive research the generic question is: "What is/are the existing characteristics of the real world relative to the specific question?" or, to use a popular expression, "Let's tell it like it is." The descriptive researcher rarely manipulates any aspect of the sample; rather he looks at it in its natural setting in planned, controlled ways and records observations. On the basis of these observations he then proceeds to describe the characteristics of interest in the population on the basis of the observed characteristics in the sample. For example, if 80 percent of this representative sample has characteristic A, then by extrapolation approximately 80 percent of the population has the same characteristic.

In most correlational studies the generic question is: "To what extent do two (or more) characteristics tend to occur together?" As characteristic A increases, does characteristic B increase or decrease? Occasionally, a researcher will manipulate one characteristic and then see whether characteristic B increases or decreases as a result of the manipulation of characteristic A. But most correlations are between measures of observed phenomena in their natural state. Some examples: To what extent do high GPAs occur in college freshmen with high SAT scores? To what extent does joint inflammation occur together with (correlate with) decrease in that joint's range of motion? There is no implication of causality in correlation, yet the typical interpretation is that if these two factors have correlated repeatedly in a sample, then they will probably correlate in the rest of the population.

In predictive research the generic question is generally one of com-

44

parison: Is treatment A different from treatment B? If they are different, is it an important difference or a minor one? If sample data suggest that the two treatments are different, which treatment is better? If the first group receives treatment A, how will that change their scores on the criterion measure in comparison to those in the second group who get treatment B? The interpretation of predictive research is almost always in terms of probability; a typical answer to its question: chances are 1 in 100 of being wrong when I say that treatment B is better than treatment A, and if that is true for the individuals in this sample, then by extrapolation it will be true of the individuals in the population. In predictive research one usually manipulates a single variable (later to be identified as the independent or research variable) and then observes what happens to another variable (the dependent variable).

Manipulation is so common in predictive research that it is often identified with it, but it is also possible to manipulate variables in descriptive and correlational research.

The above descriptions of research types are generalities based on relatively pure definitions of the three approaches. As we study each type in detail and look at examples from the literature, it will become clear that many published reports are mixtures of two or even all three types, and that within types there are mixtures of various designs. In this text we will first establish general models for each type and subtype and then look in the literature to see how individual researchers have modified and altered the designs to meet the demands of their particular question and the exigencies of their environment.

Research Design in Health Care

The biggest compromise which health care workers generally make with the ideals stated above involves the identification of the population and the random selection of a sample from that population. If one's population is all registered republicans in the United States, or all fourth-grade females in public schools in the state of Wisconsin, it is possible to compile a list (or frame) of the names and addresses of the entire population. With adequate time and financing it would also be possible to do certain kinds of research on samples from those populations, such as mail survey questionnaires which are typical of much descriptive research. In the case of the population in the public schools in one state, it might even be possible to do predictive research with cluster sampling followed by random assignment to experimental and control groups. However, when one's population is all right-sided hemiplegics in the United States whose disabilities resulted from cerebral aneurysms, it is not practically possible to identify with any precision all of the individuals who belong to that population. Given the time and financial constraints of most clinical health workers even a representative sample from that national population of hemiplegic patients is not feasible. Nevertheless, with most research on hemiplegic patients it is highly desirable to extrapolate the interpretations of one's study to the broad population. If you were working in the state of Maine and read a study done on hemiplegic patients in California, you would have absolutely no interest in that article unless there were some reasonable hope that you could learn something from it which would be applicable and useful to your patients.

Almost every research article in any health science journal will demonstrate established criteria by which individuals were admitted to the study. As patients who meet the criteria for the study come through a service, they are included in the sample and assigned to treatment groups. Data are collected, probability statements made, and interpretations done. Obviously the sample is all patients who met the criteria for admission to their study who were admitted to their hospital or department within a given time span. What is their population? As indicated earlier in this chapter, the most defensible answer is that their population is all patients or potential patients of that type who, by reason of their geographic location, have the potential to be admitted to their service over an extended time span—say, five years. The most critical question which the reader must answer for himself is: To what extent is the writer's sample representative of the patients I treat? Both psychological and social factors must be considered in answering that question as well as physiological and pathological similarities. To the extent that you can logically defend the thesis that the writer's sample is representative of your population, you are justified in extrapolating the results of that study to your own patients. In this way a clinician can learn from the literature and hopefully increase his professional competence as long as he is aware of the assumptions underlying the scientific process and the application of statistical tests.

BASIC AND APPLIED RESEARCH

One often sees these terms and they appear to have a very clear-cut meaning; yet when you look at the literature and attempt to classify research into these two areas it becomes evident that it is not a real dichotomy (two mutually exclusive classes). These terms are really the two ends of a spectrum with innumerable variations in between. This variation is explored further in Chapter 11, but for now let it suffice to briefly define the two extremes.

"Pure" research is interested in the acquisition of knowledge for its own sake without any concern for the utility of that knowledge. For example, a researcher might be interested in the effects of different types of heat on the microcirculation of muscular and connective tissue. He could pursue this topic from several points of view by performing a number of experiments, and not ever know of the existence of the field of physical therapy, and never give any thought to the medicinal uses of the information which he is gathering.

Applied research (sometimes called action research) is concerned with the solution of immediate problems without any concern for the basic reason as to why the solutions work. For example, a physical therapist might be interested in the influence of short-wave diathermy on muscle spasm in acute, idiopathic, low back pain. He might study that question and find answers, and never give a thought to the possible explanation of how it works in terms of the influence of heat on microcirculation of the tissues or on nervous tissue.

Obviously, there are a number of gradations in between these two extremes and frequently the classification of research into these two categories is of academic interest only. One important question relating to this issue is the following: Can I apply what I learned from this research study directly to patient care, or are there other questions which must be answered first? For example, are the results of Hagbarth's study of the effects of vibration on neuromuscular responses in cats directly applicable to patient care? Or would it be important to first examine the results of intervening studies which treat the influence of vibration on normal humans and on humans with neuromuscular pathologies? These questions are discussed further in Chapter 11.

REVIEW QUESTIONS

A Preliminary Research Protocol: All patients admitted to a large metropolitan in-patient, arthritis clinic are initially screened by an activities of daily living (ADL) test. Those with low scores in self-care are further evaluated. All patients with more than 30 percent but less than 60 percent of normal passive range of motion (ROM) in the elbow of the dominant arm and whose active elbow ROM is 90 percent of passive range or more, are admitted to the study. All subjects are put on the same medication, diet, and general routine. All subjects are given identical therapy programs except for the length of time they spend in daily, bilateral, rhythmic, upper extremity, active exercises which emphasize maximal range of shoulder and elbow joints. Using a table of random numbers, the therapists divided the research subjects into three groups. One group spent one hour daily (in three 20-minute sessions) on the rhythmic exercises; one group spent two hours daily (in six 20-minute sessions) on the rhythmic exercises. The third group will rest while the other groups are exercising. ROM was recorded at the beginning of the study (pre-test) and again in three weeks (post-test). The pre- and post-test ROM scores for the elbow of the dominant arm will be compared for significant differences among the three groups. Which group (one-hour, two-hour, or resting) will show the greatest gain in elbow ROM?

1. Is this basic or applied research?
2. Is it primarily descriptive, correlational, or predictive?
3. What is the population of this study?
4. What is the sample of this study?
5. What are the controls of this study?
6. How is sampling done?
7. Could other forms of sampling have been used? What changes in design would be required to use different sampling techniques?

REFERENCES

1. Drew, C. J.: (1976) Introduction to Designing Research and Evaluation. C. V. Mosby Co., St. Louis, 1976, p. 123.
2. Leedy, P. D.: Practical Research: Planning and Design. Macmillan, N.Y., 1974.

ADDITIONAL READING

Ethridge, D. A., and McSweeney, M.: Research in occupational therapy. Part I: Introduction. Am. J. Occup. Ther. 24(7):490, 1970.
Ethridge, D. A., and McSweeney, M.: Research in occupational therapy. Part II: Hypothesis. Am. J. Occup. Ther. 24(8):551, 1970.
Mowrer, O. H.: Basic research methods, statistics and research theory. Am. J. Occup. Ther. 14(4):199, 1960.

Chapter 4

MEASUREMENT

OBJECTIVES

1. *Define criterion measures; measurement; nominal, ordinal, and metric measurements. Illustrate each as they relate to professional practice.*
2. *Define parameter and statistic.*
3. *Identify level of measurement in given research reports.*
4. *Define parametric and nonparametric as they relate to measurement.*

BASIC TERMS

As stated in Chapter 1, research is designed to answer a question on the basis of collected data. The data which are collected form the criterion. The *criterion measure* is that which is measured in the study. The observations which are measured are either assigned to categories or they are given numerical values; that is to say, they are assigned numbers according to the rules of measurement theory. *Measurement* is the process of quantifying people, objects, events, or their characteristics. Theoretically, we can measure anything if the appropriate rules are used. As Hasselkus and Safrit[1] have noted: "A substantial portion of any occupational therapist's workday is inevitably spent 'measur-

49

ing' behaviors." The same can be said of physical therapists. Therapists measure strength, range of motion, motor functions such as gait or activities of daily living, temperature, pulse, blood pressure, sensory integrative behaviors, developmental level, the level of cooperation among family members, etc. They also measure performance levels of employees under their supervision, and the efficiency of the department in terms of patients treated per therapist hours, and budget matters. In order to study any of these phenomena we collect information about them and record that information as a measurement of the phenomena observed.

Some measurements are straightforward: the number of steps an amputee can walk before stopping, the time in minutes that it takes a hemiplegic patient to put on a shirt, the degree of motion in an arthritic wrist. These are concrete, observable, biological phenomena related to frequency, weight, height, time, and length. However, therapists must also measure phenomena in the psychosocial area and other functional areas where precise measurement is not possible. Such phenomena cannot be defined by specific measures such as inches or pounds; they are given, instead, a rating system of some sort. To measure a patient's independence in daily living, Hasselkus and Safrit used this measure:

> Numbers are assigned (for example, 0, independent; 1, minimal assistance; 2, moderate assistance; 3, total dependence) to the behavioral indicators and inferences are drawn with regard to the underlying property: independence.

We use similar measures with phenomena such as spasticity, motivation, cooperation, and sensation. Learning in the classroom and in the clinic is another phenomenon which cannot be measured directly; we measure something else and then infer from that measure the underlying property of learning.

It is important to be sure that the criterion measure (that which is measured) is truly relevant to the phenomena under study. This statement may appear to be obvious; however, Hamilton[2] has given a good example of the way in which we may be fooled into measuring the wrong thing.

> An example from general medicine will illustrate what I mean about the problems of the relevance of criterion. When anticoagulant drugs were first introduced as a 'treatment' for coronary thrombosis, they roused tremendous interest. A great spate of research followed. . . . nevertheless I often wondered if all that effort had been somewhat displaced. It seemed to me that the real

criterion was not the maintenance of a low coagulability of the blood, but the incidence of recurrence of thrombosis and ultimately the death rate or expectation of life. In due course, researches were published which had used these criteria, and unfortunately, the results were shown to be much less good [sic] than had been hoped for.

The attributes of interest in a particular research project must, at some level, be observable, or countable. Sometimes several possible measures are available, in which case every possible measure should be evaluated with respect to: (1) the specificity of its relationship to the phenomenon under investigation, (2) how well that measurement communicates accurately to others, (3) the sensitivity of the measure. For example, inches are more specific to a measurement of stature than are pounds; the concept of inches communicates effectively to the general population of Americans; and the inch is a more precise measure than the foot. Millimeters would communicate more effectively to the scientific community, and are more sensitive to change in length than inches.

There are four levels of measurement which are generally discussed in connection with research design.[3] They are: nominal, ordinal, interval, and ratio. Interval and ratio measures are discussed together as metric measures.

LEVELS OF MEASUREMENT

Nominal Measurement

The weakest level of measurement uses the nominal scale. In this scale the data are placed into broad categories. Numbers may be used in this scale, but they could be replaced with any other system of symbols, such as the alphabet, without changing the measurement. For example, on questionnaires where the responses were either "yes" or "no," the data are divided, and thus measured, into those two categories. In another instance, patients in a sample might be measured as belonging to either class A, osteoarthritic; or class B, rheumatoid arthritic; or class C, traumatic arthritic. The essential characteristics of the data measured at the nominal level are that the categories are mutually exclusive and independent and that there is no apparent connection.

Other examples of nominal classes are male or female; spastic, athetoid, or mixed; left-handed or right-handed; and in-patient or outpatient. There is no limit to the number of such categories. It is important to note that although numbers may be used to mark the categories—class 1, class 2, class 3—no numerical value has been assigned to the numbers. One can count the number of people or events in each category, and then state the percentage of the total sample that may be found in each category or classification.

Look at the article by Payton and Kemp in Appendix C. In Table 1, the second column ("Observed") indicates that there were a total of 60 observations distributed among the 8 peripheral nerve categories. This is nominal data with a frequency count in each of eight categories. We will return to this study in a later chapter.

Ordinal Measurement

The ordinal scale of measurement is sometimes called the ranking scale. At this level data are not only distributed into independent and mutually exclusive categories, but there is also a qualitative relationship between categories. For example, if there are 20 students in a class who hand in a term paper and the teacher rank-orders those term papers from 1 to 20 such that the first one is best and twentieth one is poorest, then not only are there 20 categories, but there is a better-than, poorer-than relationship between any two categories. In the same illustration, it is important to note that there is no equality of difference between categories, so that the best paper in the class may be much better than the second best, whereas there could be only a small difference between the second and the third best papers.

Clinicians use many ordinal scales, one example is the manual muscle test, where muscle strength is graded zero, trace, poor, fair, good, or normal with possible subgrades, denoted by plus or minus, in between. Sometimes numbers are used in manual muscle testing, 1 to 5 or 0 to 100. However, we must not be deceived by this numbering system into thinking that there is the same difference between muscles graded 10 and 15 as there is between muscles that are graded 95 and 100. It is still an ordinal scale whose "scores" reflect greater-than or lesser-than relationships; there is no equality of difference between grades. Activities of daily living (ADL) scales are another example where ordinal ranking is used. It is also important to note that there is implied an underlying continuous gradation between minimum and maximum on the ordinal scale.

Many questionnaires, attitude scales, personality inventories, and other measurement tools use a Likert scale which is generally a five-point scale; e.g., highly agree (1), agree (2), indifferent (3), disagree (4), and highly disagree (5). These scales represent an underlying con-

52

tinuum of opinion broken into five subcategories. The same continuum could be broken into a limitless number of categories, or merely divided: agree or disagree. Not only is there no objective measure of difference between numbers (1) and (2), but it is also possible that one person may highly agree and mark number (1) and yet feel very differently from another person who also marks the questionnaire (1) highly agree.

It is important to note that in both nominal and ordinal measurement you cannot perform arithmetic operations (add, subtract, multiply, divide, square) on numbers associated with those scales; you can only count the responses in each rank. Most of the measures taken in the behavioral and social sciences, including education, are at the ordinal level of measurement. This fact is too frequently overlooked by researchers.

For an example of ordinal measurement, look at the article by Carter and Campbell in Appendix C. They describe 17 tests used to measure changes in the behavior of a premature infant. All but three of these measures are on an ordinal scale.

Metric Measurement

The metric scale of measurement has a very important characteristic, namely, that the distance between any two numbers on the scale are of known and equal size. With a constant unit of measurement it is possible to assign real numbers to our observations and the data resulting from such measurement may be properly treated with arithmetic procedures; thus, the difference between 3 °C and 4 °C is the same as the difference between 20 °C and 21 °C. Therapists use metric scales daily to measure time, length or distance, weight, and temperature.

It should be noted that the same phenomena may be measured on more than one scale. For example, we may measure the strength of a muscle on the ordinal scale of manual muscle testing, or we may measure it on a metric scale using a strain gauge.

Metric measurement has generally been divided into two categories: the interval scale and the ratio scale. The major difference between these two scales relates to a zero point. In the interval scale both the unit of measurement and the zero point are arbitrary. For example, consider the Fahrenheit and Centigrade scales in measuring temperature. The unit of measurement is arbitrary; it is different between the two scales and yet both scales measure the same thing and they are equivalent to each other—there are formulas for translating one into the other. They are linearly related, but the size of the unit is arbitrary. Also, in both of these scales the zero point is arbitrary. In one scale, zero has been arbitrarily defined as the freezing point while on the other scale zero is considerably below freezing. In the ratio scale, only the unit measurement is arbitrary; there is an absolute zero. For example, in inches and centimeters the size of the unit is arbitrary although they measure the same thing. Zero (no length) has the same value in both systems of measurement and is not arbitrary. On the interval scale, arithmetic may be applied to the differences between the numbers; in the ratio scale arithmetic operations may be applied to the numbers themselves.

DIFFERENTIATING LEVELS OF MEASUREMENT

To summarize, nominal data have the property of identity; this scale identifies real differences between and among data and assigns numbers or symbols to events, objects, or people in order to classify them. Ordinal data have the property of identity and order; the data can be put in some kind of semiquantitative sequence. The ordinal scale assigns numbers or symbols to events, objects, or people in order to rank them. Metric data have the properties of identity and order, as well as the property of additivity. That is, they are strictly quantitative and admit the arithmetic operations. The metric scales assign numbers to events, objects, or people in order to quantify them.

When we are measuring strength with metric data, it is on the interval scale because no exertion on the strain gauge does not necessarily mean that there is no contraction of the muscle so that a zero on the strain gauge does not indicate absolute zero in strength. On the other hand, when we are measuring how much weight a person can lift against gravity and it is expressed in terms of weight lifted rather than in terms of the muscle strength, then we are using a ratio measurement and it is possible that the person is not able to lift any weight at all against gravity; i.e., a real zero point exists.

Most of the time, it is not necessary to distinguish between interval and ratio data, therefore, throughout the rest of this book we will refer to three levels of measurement: nominal, ordinal, and metric. The level of measurement becomes quite important when we get to the process of data reduction and also when we consider hypothesis testing through statistical tools. The level of measurement is important both for descriptive statistics and predictive statistics.

Turn to the article by Tanigawa in Appendix C. Read paragraphs 6 through 13. The measurement taken is length from the lateral malleolus to the floor. Paragraph 13 explains how this measurement is translated into the criterion measure of angle of passive straight-leg raising. Both are ratio measures, i.e., metric.

PARAMETERS AND STATISTICS

In the previous chapter we defined the population as all of the individuals to whom our study could reasonably refer, and we defined a sample as those individuals we are going to study who have been drawn from the population. It is clear that we intend to extrapolate what we find from the sample to the population. It is necessary to give these two definitions something of a mathematical slant in order to understand some of the important implications of levels of measurement.

When we are dealing with data collection, i.e., with the measurement of observations, we can define a population as a collection of all potential observations identifiable by a set of rules. For example, the rules might state that our population is (1) all adults with rheumatoid arthritis, and (2) all of the adults with ranges of motion we could potentially observe who have rheumatoid arthritis. The sample then is a subset of actual observations or measurements taken from the population. A *parameter* is a measure computed from all potential observations in a population. For example, we speak of the mean or average age of all people in the United States. This arithmetic mean is a parameter of our population. We don't actually go out and measure it even though it exists. A *statistic* is a measure computed from actual observations on a sample; for example, if we take a sample of 1000 people from the population of the United States and we ascertain their ages and derive an arithmetic mean, this arithmetic mean is a statistic.

Many statistical tests and measures, such as mean, standard deviation, t test, and F test (some of these terms will be defined more carefully later on), make a number of assumptions about the nature of the parameters of the population. For example, if you want to apply the statistical test called a t test to a given sample of data, you can only do that legitimately if the parameters of the population from which your sample is drawn meet certain criteria. These tests are therefore called *parametric*. Tests and measures which do not make those assumptions about the parameters of the population from which the sample is drawn are called *nonparametric* measures and statistics. Therefore, in general, all statistical descriptions or summaries of data and all statistical tests of hypotheses can be divided into parametric (those that make specific assumptions about the parameters of the populations from which the sample is drawn) and nonparametric (those which do not make those assumptions).

Parametric statistics require metric measurement. Nonparametric statistics are appropriate for nominal and ordinal levels of measurement. As we explore different research designs in subsequent chapters

55

we will refer again and again to the appropriate parametric and nonparametric statistics and tests. Whenever you see these two terms, you should automatically think nominal and ordinal level of measurement for a nonparametric statistic, and metric level of measurement for a parametric statistic. Nonparametric statistics *can* be applied to metric data, although a considerable amount of information is discarded in the process. Applying parametric statistics to nonparametric data is a more controversial matter among researchers. Some say that it is frequently permissible; others say that it is never permissible. No attempt will be made to resolve this issue here, but students should be aware of the controversy when reading literature. The conservative approach, however, is to use nonparametric tools for nominal and ordinal data, and parametric tools for metric data.

REVIEW QUESTIONS

1. Review the article by Houser in Appendix C. What is/are the criterion measure(s)? What level of measurement is employed? What are her data?
2. Review the article by Ayres in Appendix C. What is/are the criterion measure(s)? What level of measurement is employed? What are her data? Be sure to read paragraph 7 carefully.
3. Classify the following data as (1) nominal, ordinal, or metric and (2) appropriate for parametric or nonparametric statistical treatment.
   a. Shoulder range of motion measured by goniometry
   b. Hamstring strength measured by strain gauge
   c. Grades on an anatomy quiz
   d. SAT scores of an entering junior class
   e. Diagnoses on a neurological ward
   f. Number of therapists in each state

REFERENCES

1. Hasselkus, B. R., and Safrit, M. J.: Measurement in occupational therapy, Am. J. Occup. Ther. 30:429, 1976.
2. Hamilton, M.: Lectures on the Methodology of Clinical Research, ed. 2. Churchill Livingston, London, 1974, p. 124.
3. Siegel, S.: Nonparametric Statistics for the Behavioral Sciences. McGraw-Hill, N.Y., 1956.

ADDITIONAL READING

Drew, C. J.: Introduction to Designing Research and Evaluation, Chapter 6. C. V. Mosby, St. Louis, 1976.

Chapter 5

DESCRIPTIVE RESEARCH

OBJECTIVES

1. *Define and illustrate each of the following descriptive research designs: nominal, normative, historical, developmental.*
2. *State at least one method for implementing each design above.*
3. *Identify and evaluate descriptive designs and methods in given studies.*
4. *Describe characteristics and uses of case study, intensive case study, and survey.*
5. *Identify major concepts used to summarize descriptive data.*
6. *Critique major methods of descriptive research.*

Before we go any further into the analysis of the three types of research design, let me suggest an overriding concept which the student may profitably trace in its development throughout this and the next several chapters. If nothing or almost nothing is known about a topic, there is a general sequence of research designs which will be efficient in developing reliable information about that topic. That general sequence proceeds from descriptive to correlational to predictive. Descriptive research often proceeds from its nominal to its normative form; predictive research often proceeds from simple to complex designs and from nominal to ratio levels of measurement. This progression also relates to the development of theory discussed in Chapter 2. This concept of sequence and progression within research designs is a general one and obviously there will be significant variations from one topic to another depending upon many details of the nature of the topic and the level and reliability of what is already known. Nevertheless, it is suggested that the student keep this general sequence in mind as the particulars of each design are mastered.

DEFINITION

Chapter 3 gave an overview of the nature of descriptive research. The student might be well served to review that portion of Chapter 3 now. One of the major purposes of descriptive research is to discover some of the essential characteristics of a particular population as it exists in nature (in situ). It is assumed that this information is not readily available and therefore the researcher needs to take a controlled look at a representative sample of the population in order to observe and describe what is there.

Another major function of descriptive research is to provide some facts upon which to base reasonable hypotheses for experimental research which will generate new knowledge. Descriptive research provides a firm foundation for building new knowledge in almost any area of interest. All of the sciences which are today characterized by highly sophisticated experimental research began at some time in history with simple and careful description of natural phenomena. The therapies are in need of a great deal of descriptive information on which can be based useful hypotheses regarding the effectiveness of clinical practice.

The following are examples of descriptive questions: (1) How frequently do therapists in the state of Georgia attend continuing education programs? (2) What percentage of the patients admitted to St. Hopeless Hospital are referred to physical and occupational therapy? (3) How are rheumatoid arthritic patients typically treated in this department, and what are the results? (4) What were the most frequently used therapeutic modalities in the therapy clinics of stateside army hospitals during World War II? (5) What is the typical sequence of events in the clinical course of juvenile rheumatoid arthritis from the first diagnosis of the disease to age 25? Each of these questions are representative of one of the subclasses of descriptive research.

In "pure" descriptive research, nature assigns the treatment. However, many useful studies often have elements of predictive research, especially the manipulation of independent variables. Such studies are within the realm of descriptive research because of what is done with the data.

SUBCLASSES OF DESCRIPTIVE RESEARCH

Nominal Descriptive Research

Nominal descriptive research is the most general approach to controlled observation. It is appropriate when you know almost nothing about the topic of interest—when you don't know enough about the topic to ask more specific and answerable questions. The fundamental technique is to identify a population appropriate to your question, select an appropriate sample and then make one or several preplanned observations of that sample. These observations are preplanned because you know what you are looking for, how you are going to look for it, and how you are going to record your observations. How you are to record your observations includes an identification of the level of measurement and the measurement tool you are going to use. Frequently, the level of measurement in descriptive studies is a frequency count which is nominal level measurement. Two major methods for all subclasses of descriptive research are the survey and the case study.

The case study illustrates the general idea behind nominal descriptive research. Let us say, by way of example, that a physician refers to you a patient who has a rare disease or an unusual injury about which you know very little. Questioning the physician and surveying the standard textbooks elicits very little additional meaningful information; therefore, you decide to institute a nominal descriptive research project using the case study method. Your research question is "What are the distinctive characteristics or the distinctive manifestations of this disease or injury as exemplified in this one patient?" You begin by observing the patient carefully and making notes (both mentally and in writing) of the patient's behavior, atypical as well as typical. You may note that sometimes the patient can maintain independent sitting balance and at other times he cannot. You may decide to begin to measure the patient's ability to sit independently by doing a frequency count of the number of times he is placed in the sitting position, the number of times he maintains that position, and the number of times he does not. After a while you may decide to refine that observation by a metric measure of the number of seconds that he remained in independent sitting balance when placed in that position.

A cumulative record of such observations is given in Table 5-1. The

Table 5-1. Observations on a patient's sitting balance after being placed in a sitting position.

| | | Independent Sitting (seconds) | | |
0–5	5–10	10–20	20–40	40+
I I I I	┼┼┼┼ I I I	I I I	I	I

metric measurement of data (seconds) has been converted to nominal categories with a frequency count.

You may then decide to try to observe the patient further to see if you can determine what circumstances prevail when the patient is maintaining balance and what, if anything, occurs when he loses balance. You might in time discover that rotation of the patient's head to either left or right immediately precedes the loss of balance. And so the study continues, and in time you may have a very detailed description of the patient's motor behavior: what motor acts he can perform, in what ways they deviate from normal, a detailed description of abnormal movements, how they begin, how they proceed, and how they end, etc. You have named (the meaning of the word nominal) the essential characteristics of this particular patient; this is an example of nominal descriptive research using the case study.

Normative Descriptive Research

Let us continue with our hypothetical example above and assume that over the next two or three years you were referred nine more cases of the same disease; and let us further assume that for each of the subsequent nine cases you did a detailed case study using the same methods of observation that you used on the first one. You would then be in a position to publish a normative study based on the ten cases. In this context the word norm means average or typical. Normative descriptive research defines average or typical characteristics of a given sample. Therefore, in your normative study you would report that on the basis of ten cases you have data to substantiate the statement that 40 percent of these patients can maintain sitting balance for 40 seconds or longer if they can maintain their head in midposition during that time. You might further state that 20 percent of these patients lost their sitting balance when their heads rotated to the left and 74 percent lost their balance when their heads rotated to the right. Your data might indicate that the average age of patients who manifested this disease was 14.62 years and that the age range for your sample was 10 to 18 years. With your normative descriptive

60

research you have begun to define some important characteristics which are typical of this patient population. The methodology you have used is that of case study; i.e., controlled observation which was preplanned in terms of what was to be observed and how it was to be measured and recorded.

Therapists do many things every day about which there are important nominative and normative information which is unavailable in the literature. It has been observed that criteria for precisely defining brain damage falls into this category.[1] Similar observations have been made about the need for very basic information on the effects of therapeutic procedures, and how these effects vary with different circumstances or different patient characteristics.[2]

Earlier it was stated that two major methods of descriptive research are case study and survey. We have seen how the case study can lead to important information; let us now consider the survey. We are all familiar with a number of surveys which describe people as they are. The national census is done every ten years and describes a number of important characteristics of people living in the United States.

Let's say you wanted to know what therapists in the state of California thought about National Health Insurance and how they perceived it might influence their practice. You could obtain this information by writing a series of good questions about that topic and mailing it to a representative (i.e., randomly chosen) sample of all the therapists registered in the state of California. On the basis of their answers you could then make normative statements. For example, you might discover that 40 percent of your sample believed that National Health Insurance would increase their case load. You could then extrapolate this finding and hypothesize that 40 percent of all the therapists practicing in the state of California believed that National Health Insurance would increase their case load.*

Go back to Chapter 1 and look at the example of the two therapists in St. Hopeless Hospital. Using the survey method of descriptive research, how would you go about answering their first question: what measurement tools and what therapeutic methods are currently being used by therapists in hospitals and clinics across the country?

A check list, which is similar to a questionnaire, is also used sometimes in descriptive research. For example, one might send out a checklist of all possible therapeutic modalities to a randomly selected sample of therapists and ask them simply to check off all of those modalities which they use at least once a week (nominal data), or they

---

*The same information might be gathered in structured interviews rather than by written questionnaires.

might be asked to use the same check list and write in the average number of times that they use each therapeutic modality each week (ordinal data). From such a survey one could conclude that the typical therapist uses modality A three times more frequently than modality B, and twice as frequently as modality C. Interviews, questionnaires, and check lists are also used in job analysis studies which are designed to describe what people in certain occupational categories typically do, how they spend their time, etc. Such job analyses are done from time to time in both physical and occupational therapy and this data is used to keep educational curricula up to date.

The questionnaire is a popular tool for student research papers. One such thesis[3] surveyed by questionnaire a random sample of the physical therapists licensed and working in the state of Virginia in 1973. Some of the important data collected in this survey indicated how long the average therapist had been working, when they graduated from the school, how much they felt they knew about various therapeutic exercise techniques, where they learned what they knew about each of these techniques, how much they learned about these techniques in school and how much they learned in continuing education, when and where they took continuing education on these topics, how many continuing education courses in each subject they had taken, and what kind of continuing education they would like to have in each of the methods listed. This descriptive information proved to be of great value to the State Continuing Education Committee in planning and presenting appropriate and attractive continuing education programs for physical therapists in that state. Such papers often provide descriptive information which has a great many practical uses: justifying an increase in floor space for a department; increasing a department budget; increasing or decreasing the number of staff in a department; increasing salaries; changing job descriptions; changing curriculum; improving function and safety of equipment, etc.

Historical Descriptive Research

Historical research focuses upon past events rather than present events. Its primary tool is document analysis, which is a little bit like detective work. Historical research is always flavored by interpretations: the original interpretation of an event, and the successive interpretations of that historical document made by researchers. The major differences between historical research and other classes of descriptive research is that it describes what *was* instead of what *is*. Since it has often been suggested that those who do not know history are doomed to repeat it, an examination of therapeutic procedures that have and have not worked in the past can be of benefit to today's patients.

Developmental Descriptive Research

Developmental research describes a sequence of events over a long period of time. Classic examples are the studies of Gesell and McGraw on the normal developmental sequence of human infants. Their method employed direct observations and repeated measurements of many characteristics in many infants over a considerable period of time.

Developmental studies may also be done on adults. (For a recent example see Ref. 4.) For example, a therapist could mail a questionnaire to all newly graduated therapists in a designated geographic area and repeat the same questionnaire to the same therapists each year for a ten-year period. The questionnaire could query the development of a number of characteristics such as management skills and responsibilities, educational development, etc. That would be a *longitudinal* study. If the questionnaire were mailed once, to postgraduate therapists who would have different lengths of experience, it would be a *cross-sectional* study. In a cross-sectional study, data is taken at one point in time from a sample stratified on some important characteristics—frequently age. For a current example of this technique see Levinson.[5]

Read the article by Carter and Campbell in Appendix C. The article by Carter and Campbell can be classified from several points of view: It is descriptive research; it is a case study; and, in a somewhat limited time-frame, it is a developmental study of one child. The level of measurement for most of the parameters is ordinal, from 0 (no response) to 4 or 5 (fully developed response). Table 1 is raw data—ordinal measurement based on repeated observations.

The Carter and Campbell article is an example of an *intensive case study*.[2,6,7] What makes this an intensive case study is the number of repeated measures on the same individual with deliberate attempts to define the parameters measured in operational terms and to quantify observation at a level which is intellectually defensible. This kind of intensive study, as Gonnella points out, requires preplanning and rigorous control. Since this kind of study does not have to meet any of the mathematical requirements of predictive research, the descriptive researcher is free to follow the responses of the patient and the therapists' own intuition and insight and still continue to record useful information. A change in treatment need not damage the research design, and could even enhance it. A series of intensive case studies such as the one modeled by Carter and Campbell could lead to a normative study of tremendous practical importance to the clinician.

SUMMARY STATEMENTS OF DESCRIPTIVE DATA

A mass of raw data is often so unwieldy that it is difficult to see its important implications. Therefore, it usually becomes necessary to make some sort of summary statement about the observations made on the sample; this can be done using statistics. Table 5-2 summarizes the most common descriptive statistics for the various levels of measurement.

Table 5-2. Descriptive statistics

Level of Measurement	Central Tendency	Spread or Variability	Other
Nominal	Mode	Range	Frequency counts and percentages in categories
Ordinal	Median	Range	Frequency counts and percentages at levels (percentile)
Metric	Mean	Range; Variance; standard deviation	Frequency counts and percentages at levels

The central tendency of a set of ordinal data is the middle of the range of recorded measurements, listed in order. For example, take all of the ratings of spontaneous activity in the supine position from the table in the article by Carter and Campbell. Sixteen ratings were made on one subject performing one activity. In Table 5-3 these 16 ratings are arranged from left to right in sequence from 0 to 3. Remember that this is not the sequence in which the measurements were recorded. A heavy line, dividing the series in half, represents the median, since these are ordinal data. Since there is an even number of measurements, no number falls at the median; in this case the average of the two numbers on either side of the line is the central tendency.

With nominal data the measure of central tendency is called the

Table 5-3. Illustration of the median of a series of measures (data supplied from the work of Carter and Campbell in Appendix C)

0 0 1 1 1 1 1 1	1 2 2 3 3 3 3 3

mode; it is the category into which the most observations fall. In Table 5-1, the mode is the category of five to ten seconds because the greatest number of observations fell into that category. With metric data the central tendency is the calculation of arithmetic mean.

Let us now look at the measure of spread or variability. Say a class is given two separate exams and that the class average on both is 75. In one exam the highest score may have been 100 and the lowest 50, whereas in the other exam the highest might have been 90 and the lowest 67. In order to compare the two sets of scores we need some measure of the spread or variability. A common measure of variability for all three levels of measurement is the range. In Table 5-1 the range is 1 to 40+. In Table 5-3 the range is 0 to 3. Metric data can be analyzed with two other measures of spread or variability. These are known as variance and standard deviation. Since we are not concerned with mathematics in this textbook we will not deal with the specific properties of variance and standard deviation, although the concept of standard deviation is expanded a little further in Chapter 7.

The right-hand column in Table 5-2 is rather self-explanatory. In both Tables 5-1 and 5-3 it is possible to do a frequency count of the number of observations in each category and it is possible to convert each of these frequency counts into a percentage of the total number. For example, in Table 5-1 there are a total of 17 observations. The eight observations in the second category comprise 47.06 percent of the total number of observations. Each researcher must consider the nature of his data and the nature of the question being asked in order to decide when it is appropriate and useful to report frequency counts and percentages. Percentages are frequently useful in normative studies.

CRITIQUE OF DESCRIPTIVE METHODS

There are several sources of error which may invalidate a descriptive methodology. The most obvious are those which have been discussed in Chapter 3, i.e., proper sampling, asking the right questions, collecting data appropriate to the questions, and making proper inferences.

One major source of trouble is bias (unconscious bias, not deliberate fraud) in selecting parameters to be observed in case studies or in selecting questions to be asked in interviews and on questionnaires or check lists. It is easy for the researcher to subconsciously bias the data in directions compatible with his expected or desired results. This problem is obviously compounded if several observers are working together on a project and observing different subjects. With multiple observers great care must be taken to be sure that all observers discriminate one phenomenon from another in the same way, that they respond to the same cues, that they agree on the definitions of what is to be recorded and how it is to be recorded.

Another source of bias is the respondent who answers questions the way he thinks they 'should be answered' or in ways which he thinks will please the researcher. In some kinds of questionnaires the respondent may be inclined to answer in ways which are more socially desirable rather than the way he actually feels or thinks. People may also respond differently because they are consciously aware that they are being observed (the Hawthorne effect; see Chapter 8). It may not be possible to completely remove bias from descriptive research, particularly interviews and questionnaires; however, the careful researcher can apply as many constraints as possible, such as defining terms and methods of measurement and observation, and writing interview and questionnaire questions in unambiguous, well-defined terms which will incline everyone to read the questions the same way. Before developing a questionnaire or rating scale, one should refer to a good textbook on the subject, such as that provided by Jacobs.[8] General rules are: be precise, avoid loaded questions, avoid emotion-laden words, and, if possible, provide a series of graded choices from which the subjects may select an answer. Open-ended answers which provide blank spaces to be filled in are open to subjective interpretation and are difficult to tabulate. Be sure that the questions are ones which the respondents are qualified to answer.

A major consideration in preparing or interpreting a study which uses questionnaires (particularly those conducted by mail) is that a 40-percent return is considered a very good return by most researchers. For example, suppose that you mailed a questionnaire which dealt with attitudes toward social issues in medicine. Those who did not respond might be very conservative in their views on the matter and therefore did not like your survey questions. Without a repeat mailing your respondents would then compose a sample whose views were more liberal. If you did employ a double sampling technique and sent another questionnaire to those who did not respond to the first survey, then your second sample might be biased in favor of conservatives, depending on the questions. People who did not respond may very well be different in characteristics essential to your research question from those who did. It may be that certain personality types are more inclined to answer questionnaires than are other types, and this will bias your sample. It may be that only people who feel that their answers are the "correct" ones respond.

We have only touched on the possible sources of error in using questionnaires and other descriptive research techniques. However, the preceding information should be enough to make the reader alert to the scope and limitations of descriptive studies.

REVIEW QUESTIONS

1. Look at the study by Bell et al. in Appendix C. Describe his research design as completely as possible in terms of the classifications outlined in this chapter.
2. The following questions are taken from paragraph 1 of this chapter. Match each one with a design on the right.

How frequently do therapists in the state of Georgia attend continuing education programs?   a. historical

What percentage of the patients admitted to St. Hopeless Hospital are referred to physical and occupational therapy?   b. developmental

How are rheumatoid arthritic patients typically treated in this department, and what are the results?   c. nominal

What were the most frequently used therapeutic modalities in the therapy clinics of stateside army hospitals during World War II?   d. case study

What is the typical sequence of events in the clinical course of juvenile rheumatoid arthritis from the first diagnosis of the disease to age 25?   e. normative

REFERENCES

1. Michels, E.: Research Needs and Classical Applications: Neurological Disorders. Paper presented to the Section on Research, American Physical Therapy Association, Houston, Texas, June 27, 1973.
2. Gonnella, C.: Designs for clinical research. Phys. Ther. 53:1276, 1973.
3. Yoder, E.: Neurophysiological Approaches to Therapeutic Exercise Among Physical Therapists in Virginia. Unpublished Masters thesis, Virginia Commonwealth University, Richmond, Va., 1974.
4. Vaillant, G. E.: Adaptation to Life. Little, Brown & Company, Boston, Mass., 1977.
5. Levinson, D. J.: The Seasons of a Man's Life. Alfred A. Knopf, N.Y., 1978.
6. Frey, D.: Science and the single case in counseling research. Personnel and Guidance Journal, 57:263, 1978.
7. Sarris, J.: Vicissitudes of intensive life history research. Personnel and Guidance Journal, 57:269, 1978.
8. Jacobs, T. O.: A Guide for Developing Questionnaire Items, Human Resources Research Organization, Ft. Banning, Ga., 1970.

ADDITIONAL READING

Berdie, D. R., and Anderson, J. F.: Questionnaires: Designs and Use. Scarecrow Press, Metuchen, N.J., 1974.

Dalkey, N. D., et al.: Studies in the Quality of Life: Delphi and Decision Making. Heath & Company, Lexington, Mass., 1972.

Gonnella, C.: The Delphi Method: An Approach to Establishing Criteria for Patient Care. Paper presented to the Section on Research, American Physical Therapy Association, Phoenix, Arizona, February 9, 1977.

Kannigieter, R. B.: Guidelines for status surveys utilizing the mailed questionnaire. Am. J. Occup. Ther. 25(1): 14, 1971.

Leedy, P. D.: Practical Research: Planning and Design, Chapter V. Macmillan, N.Y., 1974.

Linstone, A., and Murray, T. (eds.): The Delphi Method: Techniques and Applications. Addison & Wesley, Reading, Mass., 1975.

Chapter 6

CORRELATIONAL RESEARCH

OBJECTIVES

1. *Define correlation and regression.*
2. *Discuss major weaknesses and uses of correlation.*
3. *Critique given correlation studies.*

DEFINITION

Simply stated, a *correlation coefficient* is a mathematical measure of the extent to which two or more phenomena or events tend to occur together. For example, if you found that erythema (redness of the skin) and elevated skin temperature tended to occur together, these two phenomena would have a positive correlation. On the other hand, if you discovered that general body relaxation and a high environmental noise level did not occur together, these phenomena would have a negative correlation. Thus, a positive correlation implies that where you see one you tend to see the other; a negative correlation implies that where you see one you tend not to see the other.

Figure 6-1 illustrates several possible relationships between two hypothetical tests; let us say that they are two new tests of sensory motor integration. You want to know (your research question) to what extent these two tests measure the same thing. It should be noted that

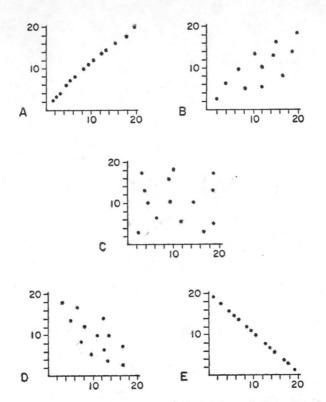

Figure 6-1. A. Perfect positive correlation. B. Moderate positive correlation. C. No correlation. D. Moderate negative correlation. E. Perfect negative correlation.

the question is phrased so that it has nothing to do with whether or not either of these tests are, indeed, valid tests of sensory motor integration. The question only asks if they test the same thing, whatever that may be. To test the question we administer these tests to a random sample of 30 subjects chosen from the population of nursery school children in a given county. When the testing is finished there are two sets of data: scores on test A and scores on test B. With the help of someone familiar with statistical methods you can apply a test of correlation to these two sets of data. Do subjects who make high scores on test A also make high scores on test B? Do subjects who make low scores on test A also make low scores on test B, etc?

There are many possible correlations between perfect positive correlation (+1.0) and perfect negative correlation (−1.0); only three of these are illustrated in Figure 6-1 which also shows the two perfect extremes. In each of the graphs in this figure, test A is represented on

70

the vertical line and test B on the horizontal line, and a perfect score for both tests is 20. Graph A is what your data would look like if you had a perfect positive correlation—each student scored the same on his two tests. The student who scored 20 on test A scored 20 on test B; the student who scored 8 on test A, scored 8 on test B, and so on. Mathematically, this is expressed as a +1.0.

Graph B is what your data would look like if there was a moderate positive correlation. Perhaps the student who made a 9 on test A made 7 on test B, and the student who made an 18 on test A made a 19 on test B. Each point then represents one child's two scores. You can see that these scores form a line which runs more or less from lower left to upper right, with some scatter. The correlation coefficient here is somewhere in the vicinity of positive 0.5.

Graph C illustrates no correlation between the two tests; one student made an 18 on test A and a 17 on test B, while another student made 18 on test A and 6 on test B. This is a correlation of 0.

Graph D illustrates a modest negative correlation, wherein the students who score high on test A tend to score low on test B. A modest negative correlation coefficient would be −0.5.

Graph E shows a perfect negative correlation; the person who scores highest on test A scores lowest on test B and so on, so that the person who scores 20 on A, scores 0 on B. A person with a 19 on test A gets a 1 on B; a person with an 18 on A gets a 2 on B and so on. A perfect negative correlation is expressed as a −1.0.

LIMITATIONS OF CORRELATION

Before we look at the uses of correlation it would be well to take a look at its major limitation. One must never automatically infer a causal relationship between any elements in a correlation. For example, one could collect data to demonstrate a very high positive correlation between the increase of cancer in the United States and the increase in the use of aluminum cooking ware.[1] One would be totally unjustified in inferring from that correlation that one caused the other although they happened at the same period in time. The naive person seeing that correlation might throw away all his aluminum cooking ware under the false impression that it causes cancer, even though the two phenomena are totally unrelated to one another. Hamilton points out that there is a high correlation between the increasing occurrence of coronary thrombosis and the consumption of fat.[1] There is a corresponding correlation between the increase in coronary thrombosis and an increase in the number of radios. A valid interpretation of these

71

two correlations would require considerable knowledge about coronary thrombosis. With that possible pitfall in mind, let us proceed to a discussion of the possible uses of correlation.

USES OF CORRELATION

The perfect correlations illustrated in Figure 6-1 (A and E) are sometimes called lines of perfect linear regression. In Graphs B and D one could draw a line which would "best fit" all the individual dots on the chart; this is called a line of best fit, or a regression line. In general, *regression* concerns the description of correlation between two or more variables that best describes the total group.

Frequently there is causal relationship between two phenomena. For example, if we were taking a correlation between intelligence test scores and grade-point average in college, we would get a fairly high positive correlation, and reason would support the idea that there was a causal relationship between I.Q. and achievement in college. Nevertheless, the correlation between these two variables would not be perfect, which suggests that there are factors other than intelligence which have an influence on grade-point average, and, conversely, that a grade-point average does not necessarily reflect a student's I.Q.

As was pointed out in Chapter 1, the researcher must produce a rational and defensible interpretation of the data.

Let's say we obtained a high positive correlation between social background and grade-point average. We probably would not conclude that one causes the other, but rather that they are both caused by other factors such as family economic status, family attitude toward education, education of the parents, and the motivation of the parents for the childrens' education. Thus, a knowledge of the subject under study is important for the interpretation of correlational data. In correlating factors A and B, at least four possible interpretations exist: A may have caused B; B may have caused A; both A and B may be caused by another or other variables; or there is no relationship between A and B.

Most correlational techniques are designed to seek the relationship between two variables. Leedy[2] lists 12 different tests in this category. Which technique is appropriate to which study will depend upon the nature of the data, specifically the level of measurement (whether it is nominal, ordinal, or metric), and whether the nature of each variable is continuous. The two methods which are seen most frequently in the literature are the Pearson Product Moment Correlation (r), which is appropriate for metric variables that are continuous, and the Spearman Rank Order Correlation (rho), which is appropriate for two variables that are measured at the ordinal level. Leedy also lists 11 correlational techniques which are appropriate for three variables.

It is also possible to apply a statistical test which will determine the probability that certain variables are unrelated in a population when one has obtained a given correlation as large as the one observed in the sample. These tests determine the significance of a correlation coefficient. Quite frequently one really wants to be able to use the statement of significance to predict one variable on the basis of another. If one can demonstrate a high correlation between pre-admission SAT scores and grade-point average at graduation from therapy school, and rationally defend a relationship between the two, then one should be able to predict that in next year's class the students with the highest entering SAT scores will have the highest GPA upon graduation. An expansion of the regression concept allows one to predict score B on the basis of score A.

Because it is possible to do a test of significance on a correlation statistic, and to use significant findings to make predictions, correlation is frequently considered to be a part of predictive statistics. However, many studies stop with the calculation of the correlation. Therefore, the author has chosen to discuss correlation as separate from both descriptive and predictive research designs.

One should be careful not to interpret correlation coefficients in terms of percentage. A correlation of .64 does not mean that 64 percent of the time when one factor varies, the other one varies. In order to approach that kind of information you need to square the correlation coefficient. For example, if the correlation coefficient of two factors is .60, one may say that 36 percent (.60 squared) of one variable is accounted for by the other one; that is, 36 percent of variable A is explained by variable B, provided that one can demonstrate in theory a relationship between A and B.

Correlational research is similar to descriptive research in that it can be used as a rather broad, relatively nonspecific search for postulates or principles upon which more specific experimental research can be built. Early in your mastery of a subject matter area you may not be able to think of questions more specific than "What things tend to happen together and to what extent."

At other times correlation may be used with a very specific and definitive question. Many tests are validated by correlational studies, particularly if you have an older, well-established test and you want to compare a new one to it. For example, test A is a well established, but expensive and time-consuming test. Test B is a quick, easy, inexpensive test. If it could be shown that scores on test B had a very high correlation with scores on test A, then one might conclude that they

73

tested the same thing and that test B could be substituted for test A. This method has often been used in educational and psychological research. A teacher might use correlation to establish the parallel equivalence of one examination with another, or to compare the equivalency of a written test with a practical test. Correlation is also used to establish the test—retest reliability of certain educational and psychological tests. For the clinician, correlational questions are more likely to be concerned with the extent to which symptoms occur together, the extent to which certain responses occur with certain diagnoses, or for evaluation of therapeutic procedures.

Study the article by Aldag in Appendix C. What variables are coordinated with one another? How are the correlations reported? How are they interpreted? What statistical tool was used to obtain the correlations? Can you think of some researchable questions which these correlations suggest? For another explanation of correlation and different types of statistical correlational tools, see Kimball.[3]

REVIEW QUESTIONS

1. Review the questions in Chapter 1 by the two therapists from St. Hopeless Hospital. Question No. 2 was: What is the reliability of "standard" manual goniometry as used by the therapists in St. Hopeless Hospital? Write a correlational research protocol for this question. Define your variables, level of measurement, etc. Make an educated guess as to the probable results. Interpret those results.
2. The fifth question from the St. Hopeless group was: Do goniometric measures of joint mobility predict the patient's level of functional ability? Write a protocol as outlined in review question 1, above.

REFERENCES

1. Hamilton, M.: Lectures on the Methodology of Clinical Research, ed. 2. Churchill Livingston, London, 1974, pp. 34, 35.
2. Leedy, P. D. (1974) Practical Research Planning and Design. Macmillan, New York.
3. Kimball, Judith G.: The Southern California Sensory Integration Tests (Ayres) and the Binder Gestalt: A correlative study. Am. J. Occup. Ther. 31:294, 1977.

Chapter 7

PREDICTIVE RESEARCH

OBJECTIVES

1. *Discuss the criteria by which experience becomes experimentation.*
2. *Define and illustrate inductive and deductive logic.*
3. *Define and illustrate type I and type II errors and power of tests.*
4. *Interpret given probability statements and relate null and alternate hypotheses to probability statements.*
5. *Define experimental controls, independent variable, dependent variable, error variables, experimental design and quasi-experimental design.*
6. *Define and illustrate one-group, two-group, and k-group experimental designs.*
7. *Give examples of experimental and quasi-experimental design studies.*
8. *Identify statistical tools appropriate to each basic research design.*
9. *Discuss design applications to research in supervision, administration, and professional education.*

FOUNDATIONS OF SCIENTIFIC METHOD

Experience

The scientific method of research is built on three foundations: experience, logic, and probability. Physicists, psychologists, humanists,

75

and theologians would probably all agree with the renowned experimental physiologist, Claude Bernard, who observed that experience is the one source of human knowledge. Every moment of our lives is experience: dreaming, driving to work, teaching, listening, reading, and thinking. Under what circumstances can any of these experiences be properly titled research or experimentation? Hamilton[1] quotes Bernard as saying that the experimental method is "experience [which] is... gained by virtue of precise reasoning based on an idea born of observation and controlled by experiment." Hamilton also quotes the father of modern statistics, R. A. Fisher: "Experimental observations are only experience carefully planned in advance and designed to form a secure basis of new knowledge." From these comments and from observation of working scientists we can see that the qualities which change ordinary experience into experimentation are the qualities of control, objectivity, and replicability.

In Chapter 3 the general characteristics of experimental control were discussed and as this chapter progresses more specificity will be brought to this concept of control. _Control_ is imposed upon experience in several ways: advanced planning of the research design, operational definitions of terms, precise formulation of research questions and hypotheses, careful identification of a population, randomized selection of samples, mathematical controls of statistical tests, and intellectual controls of logic.

In research, experience is made _objective_ by all of the controls listed above with an emphasis upon the recording of measured observations as discussed in Chapter 4. It is the measurement tool used in a controlled way which makes scientific experience objective. Precise and objective measurements permit replication of the study by others; thus, _replication_ is a characteristic of an experience which can be called experimentation. Replicability means that other people should be able to repeat your experiment using the same controls and measurements and come out with the same results that you obtained.

Logic

Earlier in this text the point was made that no effort deserves the title research unless the researcher has obtained a logical interpretation of the data in relation to the research question. One of the major intellectual tools for interpreting data is logic. Logic can be divided into two basic types: deductive and inductive. _Deductive logic_ applies a general rule _to_ particular instances. _Inductive logic_ draws a general rule _from_ particular instances.

These two processes are often interwoven in scientific thinking. One might begin inductively by thinking: If what I see in this clinic in these kinds of patients is generally true, then I can form a hypothesis of what ought to happen in all similar cases. (The thinker has gone from particular instances to a general statement. The general statement is a hypothesis to be tested.) The next step is deductive logic. If the general hypothesis is true, than it will be demonstrated in a particular experimental arrangement. (The thinker has gone from the general statement to anticipated particular instances.) Then the thinker looks at the data collected in the experimental arrangement and proceeds from those particulars to a general conclusion that the hypothesis is either supported or not supported. This last inductive reasoning from particular data to general conclusion must be based on the data alone. In the past, inductive logic was considered by many as *the* major tool of science; this is not really true. The scientific method is a synthesis of deductive and inductive reasoning as illustrated above. Let's look at a more specific example of inductive (I) and deductive (D) reasoning.

I: I have observed many patients whose skin turned bright red under hot packs. If that always happens, it might be because of the increase in arterial blood flow. (A given postulate is: arterial blood is red; see Chapter 2 for the definition of postulate.)

D: Arterial blood flow will increase by a measurable amount in areas of skin subjected to a source of superficial heat above 100 °F.

I: Set up an objective and controlled test situation in which observational measurements can be made on the rate of blood flow in an area under the influence of superficial heat. In a series of controlled observations each patient exposed to superficial heat demonstrates a measurable increase in blood flow as measured by plethysmography. Blood flow has thus been demonstrated to increase in an area to which superficial heat has been applied and this increase is significantly greater in the area heated than it was in the comparable unheated area on the contelateral side of the body. It is assumed that this demonstrated increase in flow involves primarily arterial blood at the surface because arterial blood is red. If the superficial increase were primarily venous, the skin color would be darker.

Thus, we can see the alternate patterns of thinking from general to particular and from particular to general as being essential to several aspects of the research process. These forms of logic are important for defining the research hypothesis, for defining what observations are to be made, and for interpreting the data in the light of the question asked. In the illustration above the data progressed from qualitative to quantitative.

Probability

Unless you observe every possible change of blood flow under hot packs which has ever occurred or which will ever occur (an obvious impossibility) you will take a chance of being wrong when your extrapolate from your sample to your population. You can't examine every grain of sand in the river, so there's always a possibility that some of them are not really sand, but gold nuggets. So if you examine a thousand grains of sand in a river bed and each one of them turns out to be a hardened piece of matter composed primarily of silica and alumina, you could be wrong if you inferred from that that the entire beach was composed only of similar sand. A sample of 50,000 grains of sand might have demonstrated 14 grains which were small grains of high quality gold. When you examine a hundred rheumatoid arthritics and make an observation which is true for all of them you may be wrong if you infer that the same observation is applicable to all rheumatoid arthritics in the entire world.

You never *prove* a hypothesis when your data is based on a sample taken from a population. The best you do is state the chances, i.e., the probability of being right and the chances or probability of being wrong when you accept or reject the hypothesis. The science of probability is concerned with allowing you to know exactly how large a risk you take in being right when you either accept or reject a research hypothesis. Most of the interesting questions in our world are related to the question of the composition of all of the grains of sand in the river. In most instances we cannot observe every particular instance of an occurrence. Therefore, we are almost always forced to make a probability statement based on a sample taken from an inaccessible population.

Type I and Type II Errors

Review the definitions of null and alternate hypotheses in Chapter 1. A null hypothesis says that there is no difference between two methods or treatments being tested. Pursuing our example above let us write a null hypothesis which states that there is no significant difference in blood flow between a forearm which has been wrapped in a hot pack for 20 minutes and a forearm which has not been wrapped in a hot pack. In accepting or rejecting that null hypothesis, we take two risks; these are called type I and type II errors. In the type I error we take the chance of rejecting a null hypothesis and saying that indeed there is a difference when in fact there is not. In other words, we run the risk of backing a loser. In a type II error we take the chance of accepting a null hypothesis and saying that there is no difference when in fact there is; we run the risk of missing a winner. With those two risks, what chance are you willing to take of being wrong when you either accept or reject a hypothesis?

There is an inverse relationship between the two types of error, in that a decrease in the probability of a type I error will increase the probability of a type II error for a given sample size. Therefore, if a researcher wants to reduce the possibility of both types of errors, he must increase the size of the sample. Type II errors are seldom discussed in research articles and will not be dealt with further in this text. If you wish to pursue this topic further, refer to any good standard statistic textbook such as those found in the bibliography at the back of this book.

One other term needs to be defined briefly in this area and that concerns the power of a test. A type I error was defined as the probability of rejecting the null hypothesis when it was in fact true. The _power_ of the test is defined as the probability of rejecting the null hypothesis when it is in fact false. Thus, a large type I error is undesirable, since you would want to reject the null hypothesis when it is in fact false. Therefore, the greater the power of the test the better.

Level of Significance

The science of probability is concerned with helping you to define in very specific terms what kind of a chance you are taking when you accept or reject a null hypothesis. Are you willing to accept a 5 percent risk, that is, are you willing to take a chance of being wrong 5 percent of the time, or are you only willing to accept a hypothesis if your chances of being wrong are at the 1 percent level? In statistics this chance of being wrong is called the _level of significance_. For example, look at Paragraph 11 in the Ayres article in Appendix C: "For the more accurate hand, the difference was significant at the .058 level; and for the less accurate hand, the difference was significant at the .061 level." For convenience let's drop the third decimal place and say that she is reporting levels of significance at the .05 and .06 levels. In terms of probability these statements can be translated as follows: for a significance of .05 the chances are 5 in 100 of being wrong when she says that the experimental group made greater gain in hand skill than did the control group for their more accurate hand. The chances of be-

79

ing wrong were 6 in 100 when making the same statement for the less accurate hand. These are statements which risk a type I error. Ayres rejected the null hypothesis in favor of the alternate, i.e., that treatment was helpful. These are the kinds of statements that typically appear in research reports—statements of probability concerning type I error.

There is a long-standing tradition in research that one does not reject a null hypothesis unless the probability is .05 or less. However, that is strictly a convention; note that Ayres has wisely ignored it and stated a significance level of .06. In a study such as hers that seems perfectly reasonable and acceptable. On the other hand if it were a study of a treatment where life or death could be the outcome, one probably would not want to reject the null unless the probability statement was .01 or even .001. Statistical significance of .05 or less should never be confused with "real life" significance. Statistics can give you a statement of probabilities; to interpret it you must employ human reason. Each time a hypothesis is tested and supported under controlled conditions its credibility is strengthened; that is, you can put more confidence in it. Just as you never prove the alternate hypothesis, you can't disprove the null hypothesis either, although you can demonstrate that it is highly improbable. Null hypotheses are either rejected or they fail to be rejected. Alternate hypotheses are either accepted or rejected. The fewer rival alternate hypotheses, the stronger the degree of confirmation of an accepted hypothesis.

DEFINITIONS

Experimental controls have already been defined in Chapter 3; however, that definition is worth repeating here. _Experimental controls_ are those mechanisms which so regulate or guide every aspect of the experimental situation that changes in the observed measurement can be attributed only to the uncontrolled or independent variables in the study. Because the examples of control are so varied and because there are so many aspects of an experiment which need to be controlled, it is difficult to provide a one-sentence definition of control. The student should come back repeatedly to the basic concept of control and expand his perception and understanding of this concept as he or she reads about and experiences the scientific method.

In the classic experiment one identifies a structure, function, or event to be studied; identifies ways in which its actions can be measured; then controls every other conceivable variable which can be controlled except the one to be studied. For example, if you wanted to

80

study the effect of a drug on blood pressure, you would control every conceivable factor which might influence blood pressure, administer the drug, and then measure its effect on blood pressure. In this example the drug is called the *independent* or research variable; blood pressure is the *dependent* variable which is measured. All other factors in the environment which might influence blood pressure are potential error or confounding variables unless they are controlled. In a true *experimental design* one or more independent variables are identified, one or more dependent variables are identified, and all potential error variables are subject to control. The controls are those discussed in Chapters 3 and 9. At this point in your study you should emphasize the controls discussed in Chapter 3 which are concerned with making sure that your sample is truly representative of your population.

When some of the essential controls are missing, the design is more properly termed a quasi-experimental design. According to the dictionary, "quasi" means having some resemblance to, or possessing certain attributes of. Therefore, a *quasi-experimental design* has some resemblance to and possesses some of the attributes of true experimental design. Campbell and Stanley[2] implied that that the "when and to whom" of measurement are usually present in quasi-experimental designs; what is lacking is the "when and to whom" of treatment and the ability to randomize treatments. Let us look at some classic designs, both experimental and quasi-experimental; experimental design is also discussed in Chapter 8.

RESEARCH PROTOCOL

A research protocol is a detailed plan which guides the execution and reporting of a research project. The words to emphasize in that definition are "detailed plan" and "guide". It is written primarily to assist the researcher and his associates, and is also sometimes used to inform administrators and to solicit funds from financial resources. A general outline for writing a research protocol may be found in Appendix A. The protocol is a list of steps in experimental design. When this general format is applied to specific circumstances, some of the steps may drop out and others may be greatly elaborated. For example, under step 18 "procedure," the researcher may list a detailed sequence, such as: (1) Turn on the electromyograph. (2) Calibrate the pen recorders. (3) Calibrate the strain gage. (4) Invite the subject in and have him sign the release form. Appendix B is an attempt by the author to reconstruct the protocol for the Ayres article.

BASIC EXPERIMENTAL DESIGN

To illustrate a basic research design, let us say that we are interested in studying a population which consists of exactly 5000 people, objects or events. From that population of 5000 we are going to draw a sample of 20 and study that sample in such a way that we can describe some of the characteristics of the population. How we draw that sample of 20 and what we do with it will ultimately determine our description of the research design used. There are several legitimate ways to draw the sample and to divide the sample into groups. There are also several ways in which we can apply treatments to the sample and several ways in which to measure the dependent variable. As we look at our sample and the data collection, we need to ask four critical questions.

(1) Into how many groups of individuals is the sample divided?
(2) How did the individuals get assigned to these groups?
(3) How were the treatments applied?
(4) What data were compared to what?

Let us deal with each of these questions in turn.

To answer question 1, the sample of 20 individuals from our population of 5000 can be treated as one undivided group, it can be divided into two groups, or it can be divided into more than two groups. Mathematical convention designates any number more than two as k, therefore, we can have research designs involving one group, two groups, or k groups. Table 7–1 is a summary of these basic designs.

One-Group Design

In one-group design question 2 does not apply because there is only one group which we assume was randomly selected from the population. The answer to question 3 is that each individual in the group receives the same treatment. There are three possible answers to question 4. Data can be collected once (the dependent variables measured) and compared to some hypothetical standard or norm (this will be illustrated shortly). Or data can be collected twice from the group. Typically, the data are collected at the beginning of the experiment, then the group is treated and measurements are made a second time. Thus, each subject serves as his own control. Each individual's performance before the treatment is compared to his own performance after the treatment. Each data collection is called a sample (a somewhat confusing convention). This design is often called two-related samples, own control. The third possible answer to question 4 in one-group design is to collect data from the group three or more times. Test results before the experiment begins are compared with other (more

82

Table 7-1. A summary of basic experimental designs (alternate names given in parentheses)

One-Group Designs ⟨pre/post
  1. One sample
  2. Two related samples, own control (randomized block design, repeated measures)
  3. k-related samples, own control (randomized block design, repeated measures)
Two-Group Designs
  4. Two independent samples (completely randomized block design)
  5. Two related samples, matched pairs (randomized block design)
k-Group Designs
  6. k-independent samples (completely randomized block design)
  7. k-matched sets (randomized block design)

---

than two) test results which may be measured in the middle of the experiment (during treatment), at the end (after treatment) or much later (months, years). Remember that k can stand for any whole number greater than two. This design is often called k-related samples, own control.

Two-Group Design

Going back to the original sample of 20 individuals, these may be divided into two groups and this division may occur either of two ways. We may randomly select a group of ten from the 5000, and then randomly select a second group of ten. (A variation of this would be to take the original sample of 20 and randomly assign them to two groups.) The second possible way to get two groups of ten is by matching. The process of matching was discussed at length in Chapter 3. Let us say that we want to match our individuals on only one variable, that of weight. We dip into our population and randomly select an individual who weighs 50 kilograms and assign him to the first group. We must then look through the population until we find another person who weighs exactly 50 kilograms, and assign him to the second group. We continue this until we have two groups of ten matched on the variable of weight. Some parallels to this system in clinical practice have already been discussed.

By either of these two approaches—drawing two independent groups of ten or establishing two groups by matching—we have answered the second question. With two-group designs treatment is generally given to one group and not to the other; this answers question 3. Question 4 can be answered in either of two ways which have minimal influence on research design. We can compare data collected before and after treatment on both groups, that is, we can compare the two groups after one has been treated and the other has not. Or, we can collect data before and after treatment on the experimental group and collect data at the same time on the control group which is not treated. Then the data before and after treatment on the experimental group can be compared to the data from the control group. It is also possible for both groups to be treated with different treatments (treatment A and treatment B). Either way the design is the same and the data are treated the same way.

k-Group Design

The third way to answer question 1 is to divide the sample of 20 into more than two groups. In order to deal in whole numbers, let us say that our original sample of 20 is divided into four groups of five each. As indicated in Chapter 3 matching several groups can become difficult and is therefore unusual in this design.
where each individual has an equal opportunity to be in any one of the four groups. Or, we can match the individuals in each of the k groups. As indicated in Chapter 3 matching several groups can become difficult and is therefore unusual in this design.

The student can avoid a great deal of confusion if the time is taken now to conceptualize these seven different designs (Table 7–1) and how each of the four key questions are answered in each of these seven designs. Most of the designs found in the literature are based upon these seven, or are variations on them.

It should be remembered that pre-treatment measures are not usually used if there is a chance that the pre-treatment measure will somehow alert the subject and bias him for or against the treatment, or if there is a chance that the pre-treatment measure will train the subject in the taking of the measurement. These objections are particularly crucial in psychological and sociological measures such as measures of attitude, interest, motivation, etc.

Any of these seven designs could be made quasi-experimental by removing randomization; this is the most common omission in quasi-experimental designs. This problem of randomization is crucial to clinical research, as was discussed in Chapter 3. Another problem is that of uniform application of the treatment to each individual in each group; lack of control in this phase can also reduce the design to a quasi-experimental one. These problems are discussed in more detail in Chapter 9.

Examples of Group Designs

In Chapter 1 we looked at the example of two therapists in St.

Hopeless Hospital who were interested in improving joint mobility in patients with physical disabilities. They designed a series of experiments and eight of their research questions were listed in that chapter (p. 15). We have already identified some of those questions as descriptive and correlational in Chapters 5 and 6. Let us now look at their experimental questions and classify them according to our basic designs as they are numbered in Table 7-1.

Example (1)

From Chapter 1, the seventh question was: Do the medical records of St. Hopeless Hospital demonstrate the expected level of use of quantitative goniometry? To answer this question, one sample could be drawn from the medical records and one piece of data could be extracted from each record. That bit of data extracted from each record would be a nominal level measure of the type or class of goniometry recorded in that medical record. We would have a frequency count of the kinds of goniometry demonstrated in the record. To do this we might devise three categories. The first could include qualitative statements of range of motion, for example: the patient shows improved shoulder range of motion as demonstrated by increased ease of hair combing. The second category could be semiquantitative: the patient has gained approximately 10 degrees range of motion in the left elbow. The third level could be strict quantitative goniometry: over a five-day period the patient's left elbow flexion increased from 25 to 35 degrees. Once we have gathered this data from the one sample, we can compare this to an expected level of use based on experience and/or a review of the relevant literature. We would then have an example of the first design, one-group sample.

Examples (2, 3)

From Chapter 1, question 8 was: Does goniometric biofeedback training increase functional ability? One approach to this question would be to identify the criteria by which patients would be admitted to the study; this in effect would define a population. We would then admit to the sample all patients who entered the clinic and met the criteria. We then would give all patients in the sample a test of functional ability, train them with goniometric biofeedback for two weeks, and then repeat the test of functional ability. By comparing the two sets of functional ability scores in this one group we could draw some conclusion about the effect of goniometric biofeedback on functional ability. This would meet our criteria for the design using two related samples, own control (Table 7-1, number 2). This is a quasi-experi-

85

mental design because there is no control group and we cannot, therefore, demonstrate that the patients would not have gotten the same increase (or decrease) without the treatment of biofeedback. We could have turned the same study into k-related samples, own control (Table 7-1, number 3) by giving a test of functional ability before treatment, after two weeks of biofeedback training, and a third time two weeks after training ceased. This would have been quasi-experimental design also because of a lack of controls.

Example (4)

Question 8 from Chapter 1 (p. 16) could be made into a truly experimental study by defining the criteria for admission into the study and randomly assigning individuals who meet this criteria to one of two treatment groups. Treat one group and do not treat the other group, or treat both groups the same and give only one group goniometric biofeedback training. We would then have an experimental group and a control group, two independent samples (Table 7-1, number 4).

Example (5)

Let us look yet again at question 8 from Chapter 1. Let us say that the first patient who enters our clinic is a potential candidate for biofeedback training because of decreased range of motion, and is assigned randomly to one group. He is a 40-year-old male with rheumatoid arthritis and we are going to work with his shoulder on the dominant arm. We would then look for another 40-year-old male with rheumatoid arthritis and decreased range of motion in his dominant shoulder for the second group. To increase the randomness of the experiment we could flip a coin to see which goes into the experimental group and which into the control group. We could continue this procedure over a long period of time until eventually we have both groups with a large enough n to do adequate statistical testing. In this particular example matching was done on three characteristics—age, sex, disease category. This arrangement would meet the criteria of two related samples, matched pairs (Table 7-1, number 5). Many researchers would call this quasi-experimental research because they feel that matching is not adequate control.

Null Hypotheses for Design Examples

See now if you can apply designs 6 and 7—k-independent samples and k-related samples, matched sets—to question 8 from Chapter 1. Each of these variations in design has a small but appreciable effect on the exact statement of the hypothesis and the possible interpretation of results, although all are addressed to the same general research question. The four null hypotheses for the four approaches to question 8 in the paragraphs above are as follows: (2) There will be no difference between patient scores on a functional ability test before goniometric biofeedback training and their scores on the same test after biofeedback training; (3) There will be no statistically significant differences between patient scores on a functional ability test before the application of goniometric biofeedback training and their scores at the end of a two-week training period and their scores on the same test one month after training ceased; (4) There will be no significant differences in scores on a functional ability test between patients treated with routine care plus goniometric biofeedback training and patients treated only with routine care; (5) There will be no significant differences in measured functional ability between patients receiving routine care plus goniometric biofeedback training and patients who receive the same general training, but without the biofeedback training, when the two groups of patients are matched for age, sex, and disease category.

VARIATIONS AND LIMITATIONS
OF PREDICTIVE DESIGNS

From the questions presented in Chapter 1 (p. 15), question 6 could be written so that it would be (a) two related samples, own control; (b) two related samples, matched pairs; or (c) two independent samples. Question 7 could be approached as either k-related, matched pairs or k-independent samples. In all of these goniometric studies we would be dealing with metric data.

Designs which involve measurements before and after treatment are preferable to those which make measurements only after treatment. This double-check is particularly useful when the size of the sample is small, when the subjects vary more widely with respect to the dependent variable than to the expected effect of the independent variable, and when the correlation within groups is extremely high, i.e., when there is a high correlation between measurements made before and after treatment *within* each group. When these conditions are not present it is unwise to take two measurements;[3] it is also unwise if there is a chance that the measurement taken before treatment will sensitize the subjects to the treatments or will produce a practice effect. Making measurements after treatment is most often done when psychosocial factors are involved.

Quasi-Experimental Design

A quasi-experimental design is one in which any potentially important confounding variables cannot be controlled. One of the most prevalent uses of quasi-experimental design is the situation in which it would be unethical or impractical to randomly divide subjects into treatment and control groups.

Quasi-experimental design is also used when two groups are pre-existing rather than randomly chosen, as in the case of the occupational therapy class and the physical therapy class in a given university (Chapter 3). In this instance we have two intact groups and it is assumed that the groups are approximately comparable. One is then given the treatment and the other is used as a control group. On the other hand, depending upon the experimental question, it could be that the experimenter has deliberately *contrasted* these two groups because it is believed that they are significantly different on some important characteristic. Some statisticians would say that it is impossible to do good research by making comparisons between such groups; however, as Nunnally has pointed out,[3] problems do not go away simply because they create difficulties for research. Researchers who are interested in such intact or comparison groups must simply impose whatever controls they can and be alert to the possible confounding variables when they make their interpretations. The basic question that is often asked when two such groups are compared is "Do these two groups truly come from the same population?" Under these circumstances the best quasi-experimental designs provide a control group, either an intact group or a carefully chosen contrasted group, and measurements before and after treatment.

Conine[4] has this to say about the choice of a research design:

> But the most significant problems in human sciences defy study by a true experimental method. Thus, in selecting a design, the researcher is beseiged by the sentiment for respectability and the opposing desire for practicality; one choice may restrict him to study only simple and insignificant problems, and another may put him in an inferior position with respect to the ideal design.

As a final example of research design, let me quote a report published by Pruden:[6]

A seventh grader had been assigned to do some research. When he submitted his paper to the teacher, the subject of his research was "Where do babies come from?" The paper read as follows:

Where babies come from is very important. I got a book from the library and read it, and I got my aunt's doctor book and read it. Then I interviewed some of my relatives. My great grandmother said she found Grandpa in the cabbage patch. Grandma said that the doctor brought my dad in his little black bag. And Mom told me that she and Dad picked me out at the hospital. My research convinces me that conventional reproduction has not occurred in my family for three generations.

That youngster may have shocked his teacher, but he did a lot of things right. First, he did some background reading, then some field work. Next he drew a conclusion, which his references and data seemed to justify, and he wrote up his research and turned in a paper.

STATISTICAL TOOLS

When we have asserted the nature of the population and the manner of sampling, we have established a statistical model. Associated with every statistical test is a model and a measurement requirement; the test is valid under certain conditions, and the model and the measurement requirement specify these conditions. [5]

It is beyond the scope of this text to go into detail about statistics. Siegel tells us here that each statistical test has an associated measurement requirement (nominal, ordinal, or metric) and a statistical model. We have discussed these levels of measurement (Chapter 4) and the processes of sampling and design.

Table 7-2 outlines a model for selecting statistical tools based on two guidelines—the level of measurement and the basic designs listed in Table 7-1. The assumptions of normal distribution (the familiar bell curve) and equal variance between groups are primarily basic to the parametric t and F tests. Obviously, this brief introduction has left out much detail. It may also have simplified to the point of offending the knowledge of those skilled in statistics. The author assumes full responsibility for this in the belief that it is easier to add detail and make corrections on a large, simple model than it is to build a complex model from scratch.

More complex designs, such as factorial designs and multivariate analyses, will not be discussed in this text. If the student masters the basics, more complex designs can be added to his skills later.

A model for selecting statistical tools appropriate to each rch design. [5, 8]

	Level of Measurement		
Type of Design	Nominal	Ordinal	Metric
1. One sample	chi square (χ^2)	one-sample runs	t, related
2. 2 related, own control	McNemar	Sign test Wilcoxin	t, related
3. k-related own control	Cochran Q	Friedman	F, two-way AOV
4. 2 independent	χ^2	Median test Mann-Whitney	t, independent
5. 2 related, matched	McNemar	Sign test Wilcoxin	t, related
6. k-independent	χ^2	Kruskal-Wallis	F, one-way AOV
7. k-related, matched	Cochran Q	Friedman	F, two-way AOV

"t," sometimes called Student's t test; AOV = analysis of variance.

NONCLINICAL APPLICATIONS OF RESEARCH

The most obvious differences between research in clinical sciences and research in other aspects of professional practice have to do with the nature of the questions asked and with methodology. Research in education, administration, and supervision share with other behavioral sciences some methodological problems which are less bothersome in the natural sciences and almost never a problem in the physical sciences. [7] Only a few relevant questions will be listed here in order to give the reader an introduction to these areas. What are the major supervisory problems which arise between professional therapists and assistants? Do aides and orderlies respond differently to assistants as supervisors than they do to staff therapists as supervisors? It there a measurable difference between clinical educators perceived by students as good teachers and clinical educators perceived by students as not good teachers? Will the introduction of the management-by-objectives (MBO) form of administration reduce the number of supervisory problems in a given department? What characteristics of the typical clinical environment facilitate student learning and what characteristics impede student learning?

In the areas of education, administration, and supervision, as in all other areas of research, the goal is to produce a body of knowledge—concepts, principles, generalizations, and laws—regarding behavior which can be used to predict behavior, to develop procedures and practices, and to control events effectively within the clinical situation. As with clinical studies, it is often difficult to identify an appropriate population for behavioral research and even more difficult to select an appropriate sample for study. Randomization is frequently difficult to achieve and the researcher in education and administration is often forced by circumstances to use quasi-experimental designs. The complexity of human behavior can create severe problems particularly where one cannot count heavily on the randomization procedure for the equalization of groups. Thus, it is often difficult to arrive at a cohesive educational, administrative, or supervisory theory on which sound research can be based.

REVIEW QUESTIONS*

Using the information supplied in the text, particularly in Figure 7-1 and examples developed from the questions originally introduced in the text of Chapter 1, let's look at some examples taken from the literature and see if you can identify the basic research design.

1. Look at the article by Payton and Kemp in Appendix C. Read the article through once slowly and then go back and concentrate on paragraphs 7 through 14. Try to answer each of the questions identified in the text. Paragraph 7 says that the total n was 14. In how many groups were these 14 individuals divided? How did the subjects get assigned to their group? In this study the "treatment" was lower extremity amputation in patients who were diabetic. How would you answer the question: How was the treatment applied? Paragraph 8 tells you what data were collected. Paragraph 10 tells you the standard or criterion by which the data were judged to be normal or pathological. Paragraph 11 specifies a theoretical criterion against which the actual observations of paragraph 8 were compared. With this information in mind, how would you answer our fourth question: What data were compared to what? Paragraph 12 gives you some information about the sample using descriptive statistics. Paragraph 12 also gives you some nominal measurement information about drug medication. Paragraph 13 gives you the results of the study which are summarized in Table 1 and the results of a statistical test which compared the data described in paragraph 8 to the criteria described in paragraphs 10 and 11. Paragraph 13 also gives a probability statement and interprets that probability statement in terms of a chance of being wrong in mak-

---

*AUTHOR'S NOTE—Since a good understanding of this chapter is critical to an overall understanding of the text, answers to these questions are provided on pp. 93-96.

ing the conclusion which the authors make. Paragraph 14 reworks the data in order to illustrate more clearly the specific variables about which the probability statement is made. Can you figure out what research design listed in Table 7-1 best describes this study? You should also be able to complete a research protocol on this study using the form in Appendix B. In order to fill out such a protocol, you will have to do some inferring and some logical thinking, because all of the items in the protrocol are not stated explicitly in the article.

2. Now turn to the article by Aldag in Appendix C. In paragraph 4 you will find the purpose of this study given in four hypotheses. Consider each hypothesis separately. For each hypothesis answer our four critical questions. We have already looked briefly at this article in Chapter 4. After you have identified the number of treatment groups, consider carefully how many groups are involved in the testing of each hypothesis. You will want to read carefully in order to answer this question correctly for hypothesis number 4. How did individuals get assigned to the groups for each hypothesis? What were the treatments and how were they applied? What was compared to what in order to answer the question in each hypothesis? Write a research protocol for each of these hypotheses or for the entire study using the model in Appendix B.

3. Look at the article by Taylor and Kogan in Appendix C. Answer our four questions. How many groups? How were they assigned to groups? How was the treatment applied? What was compared to what? Paragraphs 10 and 15 are particularly important; however, be sure you read the entire article before you try to answer the four questions.

4. Now look at the article by Houser in Appendix C. We have discussed this article before and you should be able to readily identify the research design in it. Answer the four questions and see if you can write a research protocol that would be representative of the work reported.

5. Read the article by Tanigawa in Appendix C and analyze it as you have the other articles.

6. Read the article by Montgomery (a physical therapist) and Richter (an occupational therapist) in Appendix C and analyse it thoroughly to discover its research design.

REFERENCES

1. Hamilton, M.: (1974). Lectures on the Methodology of Clinical Research, ed. 2. Churchill Livingstone, London, 1974, p. 19.

2. Campbell, D. T., and Stanley, J. C.: Experimental and Quasi-experimental Designs for Research. Rand-McNally, Chicago, 1973.
3. Nunnally, J. C.: "The Study of Change in Evaluation Research: Principles Concerning Measurement, Experimental Design, and Analysis." In Struening, E. L., and Guttentag, M. (eds.): Handbook of Evaluation Research. Sage Publications, Beverly Hills, 1975, pp. 101–137.
4. Conine, T. A.: Dilemmas of research in occupational therapy. Am. J. Occup. Ther. 26(2):81, 1972.
5. Siegel, S.: Nonparametric Statistics for the Behavioral Sciences. McGraw Hill, New York, 1956, p. 18.
6. Pruden, E., et al.: Ins and Outs of Research: Problem to Publication. Am. J. Med. Technol. 36:209, 1970.
7. Payton, O. D.: Research in physical therapy education. Phys. Ther. Res. 10(2):1, 1977.
8. Remington, R. D., and Schosk, M. A.: Statistics with Applications to the Biological and Health Sciences. Prentice-Hall, Englewood Cliffs, N.J., 1970.

ADDITIONAL READING

Clark, F. H., et al.: A comparison of operant and sensory integrative methods on developmental parameters in profoundly retarded adults. Am. J. Occup. Ther. 32(2):86, 1978.
Cullen, B. T., Norville, J. L., and Martin, E. D.: Management in the Allied Health Professions. Virginia Commonwealth University, Richmond, Va., 1977.
Daniel, W. W., and Coogler, C. E.: Some quick and easy statistical tests for physical therapists. Phys. Ther. 54:135, 1974.
Daniel, W. W., and Coogler, C. E.: Sampling in physical therapy research. Phys. Ther. 55:1326, 1975.
Dietrich, M. C., et al.: A Model for Work Values and Interpersonal Relations Preferences in a School of Health Related Professions. J. Allied Health 6(2):14, 1977.
Ethridge, D. A., and McSweeney, M.: Research in occupational therapy, part III: Research design. Am. J. Occup. Ther. 25(1):24, 1971.
Ethridge, D. A., and McSweeney, M.: Research in occupational therapy, part IV: Data collection and analysis. Am. J. Occup. Ther. 25(2):90, 1971.
Ethridge, D. A., and McSweeney, M.: Research in occupational therapy, part V: Data interpretation, results and conclusions. Am. J. Occup. Ther. 25(3):149, 1971.
Gonella, C.: Let's reduce the communications gap, part 4—Data presentation: Guidelines for authors (and readers). Phys. Ther. 53:871, 1973.
Lehmkuhl, D.: Let's reduce the communications gap, part 3—Experimental design: What and why? Phys. Ther. 50:1716, 1970.
Lerner, C., and Ross, G.: The magazine picture collage: Development of an objective scoring system. Am. J. Occup. Ther. 31(3):156, 1977.
Michels, E.: Associated movements and motor learning. Phys. Ther. 50:24, 1970.
Moffat, M.: Let's reduce the communication gap, part 5—Analysis, interpretation, summary and conclusions in research. Phys. Ther. 54:379, 1974.
Payton, O. D., et al.: Teaching empathetic communication skills to allied health supervisors. J. Allied Health 4(4):39, 1975.
Rogers, C.: Freedom to Learn. Charles E. Merrill, Columbus, Ohio, 1969.
Schaufler, J., et al.: "Hand gym" for patients with arthritic hand disabilities: Preliminary report. Arch. Phys. Med. Rehabil. 59:221, 1978.
Tecklin, J. S., and Holsclaw, D. S.: Bronchial drainage with aerosol medications in cystic fibrosis. Phys. Ther. 56:999, 1976.

ANSWERS TO REVIEW QUESTIONS

1. This is a one-group, one sample study. One set of data were collected as measures of neuropathy and these were compared to a

hypothetical norm which was defined in paragraph 11. This norm was based on chance; that is, if there were no pattern to the attack of diabetic neuropathy, then chance would dictate an equal proportional distribution to all nerves.

2. The total sample is divided into four groups: the physical therapy assistant group who graduated, the physical therapy assistant group who dropped out, the associate degree nursing students, and the practical nurse certificate students. Although not specified in the article it is implied in paragraph 11 that in hypotheses 3 and 4 we are dealing with the students admitted to the program and not the graduates. Individuals got assigned to groups by their admission to the curricula in question; in the case of physical therapy assistant students, they were further divided by graduation or dropout status.

The treatment applied was admission to the semiprofessional curricula. The data collected were ACT scores on admission and, for question 1, the graduation GPA formed a second set of data. Even though question 4 is phrased in such a way that you might think that the physical therapy and nursing scores were lumped together and compared with the practical nurse scores, reading the details of the text would seem to imply that these are really two separate questions and could have been divided into questions 4 and 5 so that in each hypothesis only two sets of data were compared to each other at any given time. Therefore our research design in each question is dealing with two samples.

For each hypothesis, are these two samples related or independent? If they are related, are they own control or matched pairs? If you haven't already answered these questions, please answer them for yourself before you read the next sentence. In question 1 we are comparing two scores taken on the same individual. They are not the same test; one is the ACT and the other is graduation GPA, so that a case could be made for there being two independent samples. However, they are scores from the same individuals which would suggest that they are their own control. The author favors the latter interpretation and would see this as an example of two related samples, own control. In the second question we have two groups of people who are differentiated by the fact of graduation. They are not the same individuals in the graduation group and the dropout group. We could therefore classify them as two independent samples. The same is true of questions 3 and 4: we have two independent samples, and, in effect, we are testing to see if they come from the same population. If the test for significance indicates that there is a significant difference between these groups, then we are saying they come from two different populations.

94

3. One of the slight complications in this article is that each mother-child pair is treated as a unit. Paragraph 10 makes it clear that there was one group of pairs and that data were collected from them at three different times. There is another good indication in the last sentence of paragraph 15 where it says that each pair served as its own control. The second sentence in paragraph 15 also says that the statistical analysis was applied to the scores at the three time points. Therefore, we have k-related samples, own control. Data were collected three times from the same group of pairs. The measurement tool is identified in paragraphs 11, 12, and 13. The scores of pairs on that measurement tool were studied at three different points in time. (It should be noted that in paragraph 19 there is a mention of an additional test on matched pairs between times one and three; however, that is not the main design of the article.)

4. Paragraph 7 gives you the answer to the first two questions. Two groups were formed and the individuals were assigned to these two groups by the process of matching. Each matched pair was then assigned to either experimental or control group using a table of random numbers. The treatment is identified in paragraphs 9 and 10. Both groups received a similar program of therapeutic exercise and positioning, in addition to which, during the 12-week study, the experimental group received a breathing exercise program five days a week. The contents of that program are specified in paragraphs 10 through 14. The measurement observations which form the dependent variables are identified in paragraphs 5 and 15. Therefore, we have a two related samples, matched pair design with pre- and post-test repeated measures. This is basically correct even though the matched pairs were randomly assigned to the two groups. In terms of delineating the design, the matching overrides the randomization that was done. The randomization which was done strengthens the design of matched pairs.

5. This article is more difficult to read than some of the others that you have looked at so far. Nevertheless, as a student reader you should be able to discover the research design even though some of the terminology may not have been covered yet in your curriculum. Paragraph 4 tells you into how many groups the sample was divided and how that division was accomplished. Paragraph 5 tells you the criteria by which subjects were admitted into the study prior to the division into groups. Paragraphs 6 through 13 tell you how the dependent variable was defined. Paragraphs 14 through 24 tell you what the treatments were, how they were applied, and to which groups they were applied. Paragraph 14 explains the repeated measures of the dependent variable. From this information you should have concluded that the basic design of this study is k-independent samples, where k

represents 3. Paragraphs 25 through 29 and their associated tables give you some of the results in descriptive statistics. Paragraphs 30 and 31 describe the predictive statistics and their probability statements which compare the three groups to each other. Paragraphs 32 and 33 give you predictive statistics for two independent samples where they compared each treatment group with the control group rather than all three groups to each other. And finally, paragraph 34 reports a test of correlation and paragraph 35 reports statistical tests for the significance of the correlation. Again, we see that research does not limit itself to one pure design, but uses the tools of research design in unique combinations to get meaningful answers to relevant clinical questions.

6. Here again is a rather complex paper which may require some slow reading. Paragraph 7 tells you how many groups there were and says that the control group was matched to the experimental groups on the basis of age. Paragraph 9 specifies the way in which the children were divided into two experimental groups; it identifies the standards of stratification and matching for control. The basic research design suggested here is k-related samples, matched sets, with k standing for 3. The dependent variables are specified in paragraph 12. Nominal level data are indicated in paragraph 15 and ordinal level in paragraph 16. Paragraph 17 specifies four repeated measures on the same dependent variables. The statistical analyses are given from paragraphs 23 through 26; correlation is reported in paragraph 27 and some descriptive data in paragraph 28 and its accompanying tables. The statistical tests chosen are appropriate for k-samples, either related or independent; they are most appropriate for metric data. The dependent variables used in this study are probably sufficiently well developed that metric level tests are not inappropriate. By this time the reader should be fairly skilled in the interpretation of probability statements.

Chapter 8

CLINICAL RESEARCH DESIGNS

OBJECTIVES

1. *Define interrupted time series designs; discuss their advantages and limitations.*
2. *List the essential components of sequential clinical trials design.*
3. *Apply sequential clinical trials design and time series design to given research questions.*
4. *Discuss the placebo and Hawthorne effects.*

CLINICAL RESEARCH

All of the research designs discussed in Chapters 5, 6, and 7 are often used in clinical research. Why then a separate chapter on clinical research? The special emphasis has two reasons.

The first is to emphasize the importance of clinical research in validating clinical practice. In occupational and physical therapy all research roads eventually lead to the central question: What difference does it make to the patient? The sequence mentioned in the first paragraph of Chapter 5 leads to this practical question.

Frequently the descriptive, correlational, and predictive designs discussed in earlier chapters are appropriate for answering the ultimate question of what difference it makes to our patients. However, sometimes it is very difficult to apply to human subjects in a clinical setting the traditional predictive designs which were developed in agriculture and in the basic sciences. This brings us to the second reason for a separate chapter on clinical research. There are several designs which have been developed for the express purpose of dealing with some of the problems of applying classical designs to clinical subjects.

Human Rights and Clinical Research

One of the problems we have in clinical research is that of insuring the protection of individual human rights in the research process. This is a problem of medical ethics. In recent years there have been several incidents where research did not protect the rights of individual human beings. The reaction to these reports has been an increased public awareness and demand for open accountability of researchers on ethical issues. An excellent two-part summary of the issues surrounding human rights in research has been written by Michels.[1]

When dealing with patients it usually is not possible to divide your sample into experimental and control groups where the control group receives no treatment. Sometimes it is possible, as in the Ayres study when there is no clear evidence that a treatment will help, to give all subjects good treatment according to present knowledge and then add on the unknown quantity to see if it makes a difference.

Randomization in Clinical Research

Another major problem in clinical research centers around the issue of randomization of the sample. This applies both to the random selection of the sample from the population and the random assignment of the sample to treatment groups. There are certain designs particularly adapted to clinical situations that can help with both of these problems.

MAJOR CLINICAL RESEARCH DESIGNS

Let us now discuss two major clinical designs: the interrupted time series design which takes several forms and the sequential clinical trials design. These designs address themselves primarily to questions of difference. Is there a difference between treatment A and treatment B?

Time series designs lend themselves somewhat to the study of the process of treatment as well as the product or end result. By contrast, most of the designs discussed in the previous chapters were concerned primarily with the end results. Time series experiments frequently lead to conclusions which are less generalized than the more classical designs. The major reason for this is that time series designs usually use very few subjects. On the other hand, the averaging of individual results into group means, in classical designs, often covers up real changes in some individuals. It is useful to consider time series designs as a more experimental approach to the intensive case study design discussed in Chapter 5. Let us first consider the simplest time series design, the A-B design.

A-B Time Design

Figure 8–1 illustrates the application of the A-B time series design to a hypothetical clinical study. The question for this study is taken from the questions proposed in Chapter 1. Question 6 is "Does heat before active exercise increase joint mobility more than active exercise alone?" We have already seen that this question could be answered with a predictive research design in Chapter 7.

Now, let's say we have one patient with limited joint mobility: full extension of the right elbow and limited flexion. On the first nine days of the experiment the patient receives only active exercise. On the tenth day a heat treatment was added to the routine before the same active exercise program. The measured range of flexion at the end of each treatment is indicated on the vertical column of the graph. Phase A is called the baseline and phase B is called the treatment even

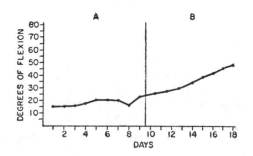
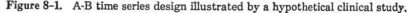

Figure 8–1. A-B time series design illustrated by a hypothetical clinical study.

though the patient was receiving active exercise throughout the 18-day period. We are interested in the effects of the heat treatment. You can see from Figure 8-1 that during the first nine days, although the patient showed a slight gain (5 degrees), the nine baseline days are best characterized as a straight horizontal line. During phase B there is a steady improvement so that over the second nine days of treatment the patient progressed from approximately 23 to 50 degrees active elbow flexion.

How can this data be interpreted? The heat seems to have made a difference. On the basis of this data the clinician would be encouraged to try again to see if indeed the combination of heat and active exercise is more effective than active exercise alone. However, on the basis of the data provided in Figure 8-1 the clinician must be cautious because there are several serious weaknesses in this design. Other influences may have occurred simultaneously with the heat treatment, so that the other factors were responsible for the difference and not the heat. One of the things that encourages this alternate interpretation is the fact that the steady rise in range of motion actually began on day 8 rather than on day 10, and the largest change between any two days occurred between day 8 and day 9 during the baseline period. On the other hand, flexion on day 9 is barely above day 7, so day 8's flexion could also be the result of chance or some transitory condition of increased pain. Maturation or the healing effects of time may also account for changes seen in the A-B design. Thus, there is not enough control on this design to make it useful, and therefore it is seldom used anymore. However, it does illustrate two very important criteria for the use of time series design: (1) the criterion measure is repeated very frequently, and (2) repeated measures must demonstrate a stable baseline before any treatment is begun. Repeated measures and a stable baseline are essential in all time series designs. The ideal baseline is either stable or moving in a direction opposite to that you hope the treatment will produce.

A-B-A-B Time Design

Figure 8-2 illustrates the A-B-A-B, or reversal, design which is an expansion of the A-B design. (A-B-A design is another variant.) Figure 8-2 continues the example of the patient with limited flexion of the right elbow. Here the baseline is established in phase A (A_1), the treatment is applied during phase B (B_1), the treatment is withdrawn during the second phase A (A_2), and the treatment is resumed in the second phase B (B_2).

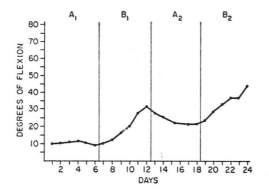

Figure 8-2. A-B-A-B time series design.

Figure 8-2 seems to indicate that the addition of heat to the exercise routine is beneficial. It is more unlikely here that some external, unrelated events accounted for the increases during the two B phases. However, Figure 8-2 also illustrates one of the problems of this design: you may not attain the original baseline values during the second baseline period. Another potential problem is that during the second baseline period, the criterion measure might plateau at a higher level than it was in phase A_1. If you have an upward positive slope during both B phases and a relatively flat horizontal measurement during the two baseline periods, you have good evidence that the treatment is indeed making a difference.

Frequently the behavior is not reversible. For example, if the vertical line represented knowledge in a subject matter area, the students would be unlikely to forget everything they know about the subject and return to the original baseline. Acquisition of skills is rather difficult to reverse. In many situations the reversal to baseline is undesirable and could not be justified on an ethical basis. There is also a possibility that factors such as patient motivation would be tied in with the treatment and account for the change rather than the treatment itself.

Time series design is useful in the evaluation of individual patients and can be utilized easily in a clinical setting without disrupting clinical routine. As in other forms of research it is important to define several factors carefully. Criteria for admission to the study (an important form of control), the independent variable(s), and the dependent variable are all important. It is generally more effective to have only one independent and one dependent variable.

The disadvantages of withdrawal of beneficial treatment may not be ethically justifiable. In order to achieve the strength of the A-B-A-B design without risking its disadvantages, the multiple baseline design has been devised. Multiple baseline design is illustrated in Figure 8-3. In this illustration we have one patient with three joints which are limited in range of motion. Throughout the experiment all three joints receive active range of motion. However, the heat treatment is applied sequentially, first to the elbow, then to the wrist and elbow, and finally to the wrist, elbow, and shoulder. (An important assumption here is that the ranges of motion in the three joints are independent of one another.) The hypothetical results shown in Figure 8-3 give strong support to the idea that heat improved the treatment. Martin and Epstein[2] indicate that the multiple baseline design may be used with a multiple baseline across behaviors, across subjects, or across settings. Three settings which might be studied could be physical therapy, occupational therapy, and the home environment. The multiple bases in Figure 8-3 are across the joints of a single subject.

It is often difficult to obtain equivalent groups among patients such as those with cerebral palsy because of the wide variability among subjects in this disease category. Martin and Epstein[2] have noted: "Because of the organic and behavioral variability in cerebral palsy,

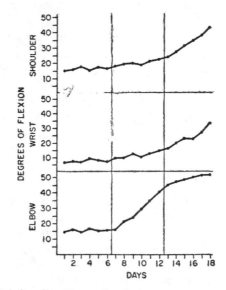

Figure 8-3. A multiple baseline time series design.

group research studies to establish the efficacy of therapeutic techniques have not been especially useful." As suggested in the discussion of intensive case studies in Chapter 5, a single time series design repeated on a number of patients which gives consistent results can build strong support for the treatment applied. The interpretation of the multiple baseline design is jeopardized if the baselines do not remain stable in levels 2 and 3 when treatment is instituted on baseline 1.

Frey[3] has gone so far as to suggest that single case designs, such as the time series designs discussed in this chapter and the intensive case study discussed in Chapter 5, are the research tools which are most appropriate at the cutting edges of a discipline. He feels that more traditional group research models which have been borrowed from basic sciences cannot answer all of the research questions important to many of us. "The simple before and after experimental group design tells us about average performance before and after some treatment but almost nothing about the individual's response to the intervention."[3] Frey sees a growing shift, at least in his own field of counseling, from emphasis on classsical research design to the simple case study design.

Both the time series design and the group designs discussed in Chapter 7 manipulate variables and assess their influence on the dependent measures. Both attempt to quantify the effects of the treatment; therefore, both can properly be called experimental. The time series designs "integrate many of the best elements from qualitative case methods with laboratory experimental design."[3]

A problem with group designs, even if they prove significant, is that the individual is lost in the group. Even in studies where treatment B is proven statistically to be superior to treatment A, there may have been individuals who received treatment B but demonstrated no improvement. Individual differences are considered something of a nuisance in most research, but they are important to the clinician who must treat such individuals. Time series designs seem most appropriate for research on individual responses to therapy.

Sequential Clinical Trials Design

This design has considerable potential for clinical questions which can meet the requirements of the design.[4-6] A question which would be appropriate for sequential clinical trial is of this type: All other things being equal (control), which of two treatments is better for this type of patient? Five things must be defined clearly when using this technique: (1) criteria for admission to the study, (2) what specifically constitutes treatment A, (3) what specifically constitutes treatment B, (4) the target behavior or characteristic to be changed, and (5) the criterion for improvement. To illustrate the technique let's look at question 8 taken from Chapter 1: Does goniometric biofeedback training increase functional ability?

(1) *Criteria for Admission*—All patients admitted to therapy during the experimental period who have less than 50 percent of normal range of motion in one shoulder. This tightness is the result of a mastectomy operation and has been present for three months or less. The patient should have no other physical disabilities and should be on no medication which might influence the results of the study.

(2) *Treatment A*—The patients will be seen daily five days a week in both physical and occupational therapy. The physical therapy program will consist of hot packs to the affected shoulder followed by gentle active stretching in all limited ranges of the shoulder using proprioceptive neuromuscular facilitation (PNF) techniques. The occupational therapy program will consist of meaningful activities designed to use the affected joint in active exercise. Length and type of treatment will be uniform for all patients in the study.

(3) *Treatment B*—The same as treatment A except that during the occupational therapy program an electrogoniometer will be attached to the patient's shoulder and the patient will be taught how to read and interpret both visual and auditory feedback from the device. In this way they will know when they are using their shoulder to its full active range. The length of time for the feedback training will be uniform for all patients in this group.

(4) *Target Behavior*—The target is range of motion in the affected shoulder in all three planes of motion.

(5) *Criterion for Improvement*—More than 15 degrees of increased range of motion will be considered improvement after all ranges are totalled. (This will become more clear when we look at the rest of the design.)

Once the guidelines above have been established, the therapist flips a coin, enters a table of random numbers or otherwise decides randomly which treatment will be given to each of the first two patients who qualify for the study. The first two patients who qualify for the study form one "little pair," the second two patients who qualify for this study form a second "little pair," and so on. For each little pair one person is randomly assigned to receive treatment A and the other to receive treatment B. It must also be determined exactly how many treatments each pair is to receive before an evaluation is made regarding the criterion measure. For this project ten treatments over a two-week period will be administered to each little pair.

Let us say that the first little pair received their treatment, and the patient who received treatment A gained 10 degrees flexion, 10 degrees internal rotation, 5 degrees external rotation, and 10 degrees abduction for a total gain over the two-week period of 35 degrees. The patient who received treatment B gained 20 degrees flexion, 15 degrees internal rotation, 5 degrees external rotation, and 15 degrees abduction for a total gain of 55 degrees in all ranges during the treatment period. The difference in total gains of the first little pair is 20 degrees and the criterion of improvement is 15 degrees or more. Therefore, the decision for the first pair favors treatment B. For this first pair we wish to record the decision that treatment B is better than treatment A according to our previously selected criterion of improvement.

We now reach one of the beautiful aspects of the sequential clinical trials design. Figure 8-4 is a statistical summary of our decision on each little pair which shows a significance level of .05 for the total project. Movement along the horizontal line is a decision in favor of treatment B. Movement along the vertical line is a decision in favor of treatment A. The starting point is the x in the lower left-hand corner. The figure is like a road map which leads from the starting point to a decision. If we cross the heavy black line (decision line) on the treatment B side of the chart, we will decide in favor of treatment B at the .05 level of significance. If we cross the decision line in the upper left-hand side

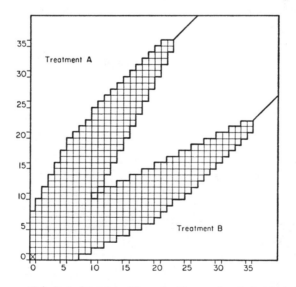

Figure 8-4. Sequential clinical trials with a significance level of .05. A hypothetical study is recorded for 6 little pairs (see text).

of the form in the direction of treatment A, we would decide in favor of treatment A at the .05 significance level. This is true no matter where we cross that line. You will notice that in the upper right-hand quarter of the form the lines from the little boxes are extended to the margin. If we cross the heavy black line (no decision line) anywhere on the inside of the form, we will support the null hypothesis that there is no difference between treatments.

Let us go back to our decision on the first little pair. We decided in favor of treatment B; therefore, from the starting point in the lower left-hand corner we move one space in the direction of treatment B and make a circle. We have moved one step toward the decision line in favor of treatment B. Let us assume that our next little pair decides in favor of treatment A. We would move one space *from our last decision* in the direction of treatment A and make a mark. Let us assume that our third little pair did not reach a criterion of significant difference, that there was only a 7-degree difference between the gain of the person receiving treatment A and the gain of the person receiving treatment B. That little pair is not recorded at all. According to Figure 8–4, the next three decisions were in favor of treatment B and so our circles move in a straight line toward the B decision line. The reader can see that if we continue with our pairs and decisions long enough we would eventually cross one of the heavy black lines. This could happen after we have recorded 8 pairs if we moved in one straight line. On the other hand, it could take as many as 58 pairs in order to reach a decision in favor of either treatment, or to exit into the no-significance space in the middle. We could reach the no-significance area in as little was 20 moves. Figure 8–4 has been drawn as the .05 level of significance. It is possible to obtain forms for the .01 level of significance, and there are also mathematical formulae for deriving other significance levels.

Advantages of Sequential Trials Design

The beauty of this design lies in the fact that all the mathematical and statistical formulae have been worked into the form, and that it allows us to take the patients as they appear in the clinic, two at a time, and work with them so that one does not need to identify his sample ahead of time. This is an important factor for clinical research because very rarely can the clinician identify a sample of 30 or more patients and randomly divide them into two groups to fit a more traditional research design. But with sequential trials you can—over a period of years if necessary—identify a sample of 60 patients, two at a time, and randomly divide them into two groups. Another major advantage of sequential trials which is particularly appropriate to clinical studies is that as soon as you reach the level of significance you can stop the experiment. You do not have to collect data on 30 patients and then do your statistical tests and discover that you might have been able to reach a significant outcome in half the time. If our hypothetical case in Figure 8-4 turned out to favor treatment B after 8 pairs, you could then stop the experiment and begin to give all of your patients the preferred treatment. You could then begin a new experiment comparing treatment B to another treatment.

There are many important questions in occupational and physical therapy which are yet unanswered. So much of what we do is based on the "conventional wisdom" of the profession, i.e., word of mouth and empirical case reports. As noted in Chapter 1, no one is in a better position to demonstrate the validity of clinical practice than the practicing clinicians. Given a certain modality (very broadly defined as anything done for the purpose of altering patient behavior), what are its physiological or psychological effects on normals? What are its physiological effects on patients, that is, how does pathology change the physiological effects of the modality? If pathology does change the physiological effects, under what circumstances and with what dosages, and with what pathology does it change them? What are the effects of changing the dosage, the frequency, the duration, the intensity of any given modality of treatment? What is the purpose of using this modality in this particular case and what normative data base does this case contribute to? What are the side effects of this modality at this dosage, frequency, duration, or intensity? Given the above information on any two modalities, how do the answers change when the two are applied concurrently? How do they interact and influence one another? If someone walked into a clinic where you were working and asked the questions listed above concerning a certain modality which you were applying to any patient, what valid information could you supply as answers?

For all its intuitive appeal, clinical trials design has been little used in published literature. For an example* see Gault.[7]

PLACEBO EXPERIMENTS

The reader may already be familiar with the concept of a placebo. In traditional pharmaceutical research the placebo is an inactive substance which is usually shaped and colored to look like the active drug being studied. It is given to a control group to test the

---

*Thanks to Dr. Pamela Catlin of Emory University for calling this reference to my attention.

therapeutic effects of the active drug. The patients never know which drug they are getting—the active or the inactive one. Frequently the researchers use a double blind procedure where no one knows who is getting the placebo and who is getting the drug except one person who, ideally, has no other connection with the study except to dispense the two medications. If the active drug is no more effective than the placebo, it is generally discarded as a therapeutic tool. However, Benson and Epstein[8] have written a fascinating article on how the placebo alone can be used for therapeutic purposes.

HAWTHORNE EFFECT

A concept which is clearly distinct from placebo and yet related in therapeutic theory is that of the Hawthorne effect. The Hawthorne effect derives its name from a study done by Elton Mayo and a group of researchers from Harvard University at the Hawthorne factory of the Western Electric Company between 1927 and 1932.[9] They originally started out to study the effect of lighting on fatigue and efficiency in factory workers. However, as the study progressed they soon discovered that no matter what they did to the lighting, production went up and the workers reported being less tired. As research in factory lighting it may have been a failure, but Mayo and his workers recognized an important ramification. In a series of subsequent experiments they were able to demonstrate that the workers' *knowledge* that they were participating in an experiment significantly changed their perceptions of the job situation and improved their productivity. The experiment became one of the classic studies in motivation, demonstrating the beneficial effects of being made to feel important and different in the work setting.

Clearly, the Hawthorne effect could operate in a clinical research study. If the patients know that they are participating in a research study, they may be motivated to perform better so that their improvements are in part due to the study itself and not necessarily the treatment. With the emphasis today on human rights and informed consent, it is almost impossible to do a clinical study in which patients do not know that they are participating in a study; a release form is usually required by law. Therefore, the clinical researcher must be ever aware of the Hawthorne effect which, like the placebo, may be a powerful tool for therapeutic improvement. Perhaps the best one can do is to try to make the Hawthorne effect equally effective on all patients involved in the study.

REVIEW QUESTIONS

Unfortunately a fairly thorough review of occupational and physical therapy literature revealed no sample of time series design or sequential clinical trials. The reader therefore is alerted to the possibility of doing something new, creative, and important for professional development by applying these designs to clinical questions and publishing their results. To prepare for such an undertaking consider the following questions.

1. In the text we looked at question 6 from Chapter 1: Does heat before active exercise increase joint mobility more than active exercise alone?, and developed time series designs around it. Now, take the question and develop a sequential clinical trials protocol for that question.
2. In the text we looked at question 8 from Chapter 1: Does goniometric biofeedback training increase functional ability?, and developed clinical sequential trials with it. Now, take the question and develop several time series experiments with it.
3. How might the placebo and/or Hawthorne effects influence the studies which you designed in questions 1 and 2 above?

REFERENCES

1. Michels, E.: Research and human rights: part 1. Phys. Ther. 56:407; part 2: 546, 1976.
2. Martin, J. E., and Epstein, L. H.: Evaluating treatment effectiveness in cerebral palsy: single-subject designs. Phys. Ther. 56:285, 1976.
3. Frey, D.: Science and the single case in counseling research. Personnel and Guidance Journal 57:263, 1978.
4. Bross, I.: Sequential medical plans. Biometrics 8:189, 1952.
5. Armitage, P.: Sequential Medical Trials. Charles C Thomas, Springfield, Ill., 1960.
6. Gonnella, C.: Designs for clinical research. Phys. Ther. 53:1276, 1973.
7. Gault, S. J., and Spyker, J. M.: Beneficial effect of immobilization of joints in rheumatoid and related arthritides: A splint study using sequential analysis. Arthritis Rheum. 12:34, 1969.
8. Benson, H., and Epstein, M. D.: The placebo effect: A neglected asset in the care of patients. JAMA 232 (12) 1225, 1975.
9. Todes, J. L., et al.: Management and Motivation: An Introduction to Supervision. Harper and Row, N.Y., 1977.

ADDITIONAL READINGS

Anton, J. L.: Intensive experimental designs: A model for the counselor/researcher. Personnel and Guidance Journal 57:273, 1978.
Bull, J.: The historical development of clinical therapeutic trials. Chronic Dis. 10:218, 1959.
Chassan, J.: Research Design in Clinical Psychology and Psychiatry. Appleton-Century-Crofts, New York, 1967.

Davidson, P., and Costello, C.: N = 1: Experimental Studies of Single Cases. Van Nostrand, New York, 1969.

Drew, C. J.: Introduction to Designing Research and Evaluation. C. V. Mosby, St. Louis, 1976.

Glass, G. V., et al.: Design and Analysis of Time Series Experiments. Colorado Associated University Press, Boulder, Colo., 1976.

Hersen, M., and Barlow, D.: Single Case Experimental Designs: Strategies for Studying Behavior Change. Pergaman Press, New York, 1976.

Chapter 9

VALIDITY AND RELIABILITY

OBJECTIVES

1. *Define validity in relation to research design and discuss its relevance.*
2. *Define reliability and relate it to research design.*
3. *Define internal validity and external validity; give several examples of threats to each.*
4. *Identify validity and reliability data presented in given studies.*
5. *Define the following types of test validity: face, content, construct, concurrent, predictive.*
6. *Discuss methods of evaluating the validity and reliability of tests, standard error, measurement tools, research questions, and research designs.*

VALIDITY

The word validity has been used throughout this book. The reader should already have the clear working concept of validity as meaning—appropriateness, truthfulness, supportableness. The purpose of this chapter is to expand on this fundamental definition and discuss some of its major implications.

A test in anatomy is valid if it gives a true indication of the student's

111

knowledge of anatomy. A personality test is valid if it accurately reflects the extent to which a person possesses certain characteristics. A measurement tool is never just valid; it is valid for making a particular measurement. A ruler is a valid instrument for measuring length, distance or circumferences; it is not a valid instrument for measuring weight. In exactly the same sense, a research design is never valid in itself, it is only valid for testing a particular question.

Crocker[1] defines validity as "the extent to which measurements are useful for making decisions relevant to a given purpose." Questions of validity are first and foremost questions of logic and rationality; there are many instances when mathematical tools can be brought to the assistance of reason, but they can never be substituted for it. The question of validity can be attached to every single item on the research protocol in Appendix B. Is this question a valid one? Will its answer give me useful information of the type that I want or need? Given a valid question, are the data that I plan to collect valid for answering that question? Is the criterion measure suitable for answering the question? Is the measurement tool chosen appropriate to the criterion? Is the statistical tool appropriate to the level of measurement and to the way the question is phrased? If any point in the research protocol is invalid, then the entire study is in jeopardy.

RELIABILITY

At this point the reader also has an intuitive grasp of the word reliability as meaning stability, repeatability, dependability. Reliability is most important where criterion measures and measurement tools are concerned. If a measuring tape is made of highly elastic material so that every time you apply it to one edge of a table you get a measurement of different length, then that measurement tool is highly unreliable. If you have a table that is exactly 3 feet wide, a hundred different people should be able to measure it with the same tape measure and come out with exactly the same answer each time if the tape measure has a high degree of reliability. Any variability in 100 such measurements should be attributable to human error rather than error in the measuring device. If the valid anatomy quiz is also reliable, then the students should make exactly the same score on the quiz the second time they take it as they did the first time, assuming that they learn nothing during the period between the two tests. If a personality test is reliable, then changes in scores over time should indicate a change in the personality. The more unreliable the test, the less you can depend upon the results as a guide to action.

By way of example, let us suppose that a rifleman fires 100 rounds at a bull's-eye type target. If every bullet hits the target, but in a hundred different places scattered all over the target, his marksmanship is valid but not reliable. If all 100 bullets enter a circle 3 inches in diameter (the same size as the bull's-eye), but that circle is in the upper left-hand-corner of the target, his marksmanship is reliable but without validity. If all hundred bullets enter the bull's-eye, his marksmanship has both validity and reliability. The point here is that it is possible to have one without the other.

INTERNAL AND EXTERNAL VALIDITY

In discussing internal and external validity in research design, most writers refer to Campbell and Stanley[2] as the standard text on this subject. According to Campbell and Stanley, internal validity is an absolute minimum without which the experiment cannot be interpreted. Internal validity refers to the relationship between the independent and the dependent variables. A study is *internally valid* when the differences which are measured in the dependent variable are accounted for by differences in the independent variables. Any threat to internal validity represents a loss of control over that relationship which results in a loss of technical soundness in the study. The major means of maintaining internal validity are the controls discussed in Chapter 3. Threats to internal validity are threats to the conclusion that any change demonstrated in the dependent variable is accounted for by changes in the independent variable. A study has high internal validity when all factors which might influence the dependent variable are controlled except the variables under study.

External validity is concerned with the generalization from the sample to the population; therefore, methods of sampling are crucial. The more externally valid the study, the more safely one can make predictive statements about the population on the basis of the results of the study.

Threats to Internal Validity

Campbell and Stanley[2] discuss eight threats to internal validity: history, maturation, testing, instrumentation, statistical regression, bias in sampling, experimental mortality and selection interaction. Let us discuss each one of these briefly.

History

History refers to the passage of time and/or concurrent experience which can change the outcome of a study. Several designs are particularly vulnerable to this problem: the before/after measurement design, repeated measures, and the time series design. For example, if you use the before/after test design with no controls and you say that the patients got better as a result of your treatment, it could be that the natural history of the disease caused them to get better rather than your treatment, or that mere passage of time may have produced the changes seen. On the other hand, developmental studies are so designed that history is the independent variable.

Maturation

Maturation is a special form of history. In addition to age it includes things like growing wiser or growing more tired. When dealing with human subjects and affective materials, even something as little as a good or bad weekend experience may be a history which confounds your variables if your before and after tests are done on Friday and Monday. The two major controls for history and maturation are randomization and control groups. Control groups are particularly powerful against these two threats to internal validity. Randomization takes care of systematic influences by spreading the influences of history and maturation equally among all groups. In the time series design, the A-B-A-B design is intented to help control for the variable of maturation or history.

Repeated Testing

Repeated testing is, obviously, a primary threat in repeated measures designs. A person may learn something about the test itself when taking it the first time which allows him to make a better score when taking the test the second time, even though there has been no improvement in the characteristic being measured. The effects of learning how to do the test could easily influence the results when one is using tests like manual muscle testing, vital capacity, and activities of daily living (ADL) testing. In using a strain gage or an unfamiliar functional test it may make sense to let your subjects practice a test until they learn how to do it, then ask for their maximum effort.

Instrumentation

Instrumentation refers to changes in calibration, such as the elastic tape measure, which can distort results. The same threat is present with observational measures if the observers change the way in which they observe and record their observations. This is a common source of internal invalidity when judgment on the part of the observer is required, as in the rating scales used by Carter and Campbell (Appendix C) or in manual muscle testing. Human observers are much more likely to get out of calibration than are mechanical contrivances or instruments. One useful control for this problem is replication, that is, measuring several times and then averaging the results. Multiple observers is another available control if one is dealing with human measuring instruments rather than mechanical. When human observers are rating data, an approach to dealing with grader bias is to shuffle the before and after test data so that the observer does not know where the data came from and therefore will not be biased.

Statistical Regression

Statistical regression is particularly threatening when groups have been formed on the basis of extreme scores. For example, one might establish two experimental groups where one group is, by definition, individuals who score high on an IQ test and the second group is formed by individuals who fall in the middle range of an IQ test. Statistical regression would almost guarantee in this case that the subjects classified on the basis of their extreme score would regress toward the middle. Regression here means movement towards the average or mean, and is likely to happen in repeated measures to those individuals who have atypically high or atypically low scores. In such cases changes on the second test may be the result of statistical regression rather than actual change in behavior.

Bias

Bias results from differential selection of group members. In true experimental designs one sample is drawn from the population and then individuals are randomly assigned to groups. However, in quasi-experimental designs it is often not possible to do this and the groups are formed in some other way. For example, groups may be based on pre-existing conditions, such as two therapy classes designated as an experimental group and a control group. Under these conditions it is likely that a bias has been introduced into the research. The same might be true if a certain ward in a hospital is designated as an experimental group and another ward as the control group. One way of dealing with this threat is to use matched pairs. However, as we have seen earlier, this is not always an effective method of control since it can introduce biases of its own.

Experimental Mortality

Experimental mortality refers to a differential loss of subjects from the groups. Mortality here means dropping out of the experiment. Subjects may fail to show up the day that you are doing testing, and it may be that some extraneous factor is operating to differentially select the subjects who drop out of the study. This extraneous bias may influence your results. In the chapter on questionnaires and surveys we saw that subjects may differentially drop out of your study on the basis of their reaction to your questions. Follow-up investigations are particularly threatened by this problem. The Hawthorne effect discussed in Chapter 8 might also be considered a threat to internal validity because the experimental group is made to feel special and that perception alters their responses.

Selection Interaction

Selection interaction is most likely to occur when there is no control group or when the control group is not equivalent to the experimental group. In such cases the factors which led to selection of the experimental group may interact with maturation or history or testing; this interaction may cause change rather than your treatment. For example, the experimental group is the junior occupational therapy class, the control group is the senior occupational therapy class; the dependent variable is a perceptual motor test administered repeatedly using a before and after test design. The independent variable could be training in a novel motor task. A greater improvement in the junior class could be attributed to an interaction between the selection process (junior versus senior) and maturation (the seniors have already had the junior curriculum which includes instruction in perceptual-motor disabilities which the juniors haven't had). With these two groups training in the novel motor task may thus have no significant influence on the perceptual motor test scores.

Threats to External Validity

Campbell and Stanley list four threats to external validity. They are reactive or interaction effects of testing, interaction effects of selection biases, reactive effects of experimental arrangement, and multiple treatment interference. Remember that according to our definition of external validity, these are threats to the representativeness of your sample which in turn threatens the validity of inference or prediction to population characteristics or behavior.

Interaction Effects of Testing

Interaction effects of testing are related to the internal threat, repeated testing. However, here we are considering the possibility that in the process of taking and reacting to the tests, the sample may become different in some important way from the population which they are supposed to represent. This would be likely to occur when the test instrument is something that the subject must practice with before you could get a reliable score. An example is vocational testing. This factor should always be considered when an experimenter is interpreting his results and projecting those results onto the population.

Selection Biases and Experimental Arrangements

These external threats are not often encountered in physical and occupational therapy research; they are sometimes a problem in certain areas of psychological research.

Multiple Treatment Inference

This threat to external validity refers to designs where there are more than one experimental or independent variable. In such cases the interaction between the experimental variables can confuse the results.

No experiment is ever perfect such that every internal and external threat to validity is avoided. In fact, quite frequently external validity and internal validity war against one another and the researcher has to make trade-offs between the two in order to get the best feasible arrangement. At one point in his research the experimenter may wish to emphasize the precision of his results and may therefore sacrifice some degree of external validity. At another point of his research the researcher may wish to emphasize the applications of his study to the world beyond the laboratory and may therefore make some sacrifices of internal validity in order to achieve more predictability. The researcher is faced with the practical decision of doing nothing because it can not be done perfectly, or doing the best he or she can within the confines of the environment in which the research must be done. Again, practicality and careful thinking about what it is you are trying to accomplish are keys to good research.

117

TYPES OF TEST VALIDITY

Test makers in the psychosocial sciences, particularly psychology and education, often speak of several different types of validity. These types include face, content, construct, concurrent, and predictive. Given that the validity of a measurement tool is defined as the extent to which that tool measures what it claims to measure, what are the uses of validity? Valid data are useful in that they enable the experimenter to make some true inferences from the results of using the measurement instrument. We will relate this use to content and construct validity. Another measured use of validity data is the prediction of some aspects of behavior in situations other than the one in which the measurements were taken. We will relate to this purpose in the discussion of concurrent and predictive validity. In general, validity is determined by comparing performance on the tests to other objective and independently observable facts about the behavior of interest.

Face Validity

Face validity relates to the subject's acceptance of the test. In some ways it is the public relations aspect of test giving. Patients will sometimes resist taking a test if it doesn't "make sense to them," that is, if it doesn't appear to be related to something they can understand and accept. For example, compare and contrast the vital capacity test as a measure of lung function and the frog test as a measure of pregnancy. The first test has clear face validity, blowing into a tube and measuring the amount of air that one can expire in one breath is clearly related to lung function. But only an endocrinologist could immediately understand the validity of the frog test; it therefore has no face validity for the average person. Face validity can be important in winning a patients' cooperation in a test. On the other hand there are times when the experimenter may not want any face validity in the test because he may wish to disguise the purpose of the test in order not to bias the subject's answers. In choosing a test, therefore, some thought should be given to the validity of its appearance and to the usefulness of that appearance.

Content Validity

Content validity raises the questions "Does this measure represent what I am interested in?" "Does it truly sample the behavior that I am interested in?" "Does it truly represent what I want to measure?" Content validity may deal with content in the usual sense of factual information or it may deal with process, such as manual dexterity. The scope of a given test should be proportional and comprehensive. It should be proportional in the same sense in which we talked about proportionality in stratified sampling. For example, a comprehensive test in anatomy should have a proper proportion of questions dealing with gross anatomy, neuroanatomy, and histology.

Construct Validity

Construct validity is related to content validity, but it is more abstract. Constructive validity involves all the other types of validity. It addresses the questions "What does the score on this test mean or signify?" "What does it tell us about the person, object, or characteristic being measured?" Construct validity is related to the concept of hypothetical constructs which were discussed in Chapter 2. The presence of construct validity in a test grounds that test behavior in theory. Construct validity is particularly important when we are measuring hypothetical constructs such as intelligence, spacial relationships, verbal reasoning, concept formation, motor abilities, and figure-ground differentiation. Because it is tied so clearly to behavior, construct validity shades into the next two types of validity which are criterion referenced.

Concurrent Validity

Concurrent validity refers to the relationship between test scores (or other measures) and "criterion states" or other measures where validity is known. The word concurrent implies clearly that this relationship exists at approximately the same time a test is given. We discussed criterion measures in Chapter 4. Here criterion refers to an external standard which is either met or not met. Either a student can correctly test the strength of the biceps muscle or he cannot. The patient can either lift a weight a given distance in a given position or he cannot. A student can either name every muscle in the upper extremity or she cannot. An example of this type of concurrent validity testing would compare the manual muscle test to testing strength with the dynamometer. Either the two are comparable or they are not. One may also express the extent to which one is comparable to the other.

Most frequently, concurrent validation is used to establish the validity of a new test in comparison to an older test for which the validity is known. For example, a new IQ test which is quick and inexpensive could be compared to the well-established Stanford-Binet or

Wexler-Belview tests. A paper and pencil personality test could be compared to the Rorschach; the Bennett Dexterity Test could be compared to a current job performance test. Concurrent validity may sometimes be used as a stepping stone to the development of predictive validity. How well is George functioning today on the basis of an ADL test? This would be a current question. On the basis of an ADL test, can we predict that George will become more functional at some time in the future? This would be a question of predictive validity.

Predictive Validity

Predictive validity is future-oriented on the basis of a measure made today. Does the score on the ADL test today predict the patient's future functional ability? Predictive validity is also criterion-related; it is related to outside objective criteria or direct measures of performance. As in the discussion of criterion measures in Chapter 4, it is important to be sure that the criterion to which the test is correlated is the correct one. If a test or measure is predictively valid, then we can say that people who do well on the test will probably achieve later at a specific level. An example: Students with scores above a certain level on this test are much more likely to be successful at verbal tasks than they are at manual tasks.

STANDARD ERROR

Let us return for a moment to the subject of reliability. If we were to measure the heights of 50 people, there would be two sources of variability, real variance in actual heights of the subjects and error variance in the measurement tool. Variance is a measure of variability. A reliable measurement tool is one where the variance due to error is small in comparison to the variance due to real differences in the objects measured. The best test for reliability is repeated measures of the same object with the same instrument. This is relatively easy to do with physical and biological measures, and much more difficult to do with psychological measures where the subject may change as a result of the testing procedure.

If you took many measures of one person's height, you would get a distribution of measures. At a practical level the true height can be defined as the mean or average of all of the heights measured. The standard deviation of all of those measures is called the *standard error* of measurement. Nineteen times out of twenty, the true score will lie within two standard errors of the mean. Note that this standard error refers to measurements taken from one individual. *Sampling error* is concerned with the error of measurements on different individuals. In evaluating a test one should look at the reliability coefficient which we will talk about shortly. In evaluating individual scores one should take account of the standard error.

USING CORRELATION COEFFICIENTS

The primary tool for establishing both validity and reliability of tests and measurement tools is the technique of correlation which was discussed in Chapter 6. Validity and reliability data are published and reported in the form of correlation coefficients which vary between 1.0 and −1.0. These validity and reliability coefficients are given the same interpretation as are other correlation scores. The closer the validity or reliability coefficient is to 1.0, the more reliable and more valid is your instrument. We are speaking now of reliability, concurrent validity, and predictive validity. Face, content, and construct validity are more frequently established descriptively by panels of appropriate experts. The same is true of the validity and reliability of research questions and research designs; these are established primarily by rational thinking.

You will probably never see a reliability or validity coefficient for any test exactly at the 1.0 level. On the other hand, if validity and reliability data fall below .5, one should be cautious about the interpretation of measurement results. Whether a coefficient between .5 and 1.0 is acceptable or not depends upon what you are going to do with the data. The more important the decision, the higher validity and reliability should be.

Validity and reliability data of test measures are seldom reported in journal articles. One reason is space limitations; a second reason is that the writer frequently makes assumptions about the sophistication of the reader and assumes that if the reader is truly interested in the material being reported, he is either already familiar with the background or will make the effort to become familiar with it. For example, in paragraph 7 where Ayres reports on the measurement instrument used in her study, the Motor Accuracy Test of the Southern California Sensory Integration Test, she gives only a reference to the test manual (her reference 4). The reader, not already familiar with this test, can refer back to the test manual which will probably include several pages of validity and reliability data including a description of the sample on which the test was validated, the population to which that sample belonged, the number of people involved, and the exact procedures for establishing the validity and reliability coefficients. Look at paragraph 11 in the article by Tyler and Kogan and paragraph 12 in the article by Montgomery and Richter in Appendix C. What do they have to say about the validity and reliability of the test they used?

Crocker[2] discusses validity and reliability and then uses these concepts to evaluate the Field Work Performance Report and the Certification Examination which are used to validate the education of occupational therapy students. She concluded that the Field Work Performance Report has good content and concurrent validity but poor predictive validity. The Certification Examination has good content validity and poor predictive validity, and its concurrent validity is questionable. Neither measure has been assessed for construct validity. Her discussion is an excellent example of the uses of these concepts.

For validity and reliability data on hundreds of different psychological, vocational, aptitude, and interest tests, see Buros.[3]

REVIEW QUESTIONS

1. If you have read this book straight through and done all of the review questions and work suggested, you should have in your possession several research protocols which you have written. Go back and review each of those protocols now. Can you identify any potential threats to internal or external validity? What is the validity and reliability of your dependent variable? How do you know? If you feel that you are lacking information on the validity and reliability of your criterion measure, how could you find information about its validity and reliability? Return to this question again after you have read Chapter 10.
2. Reread the article by Houser in Appendix C. If you were going to repeat this study exactly as Houser did it, what would you identify as your controls against internal invalidity? What controls might you establish for assuring the validity and reliability of the dependent variables which are identified in paragraph 5?

REFERENCES

1. Crocker, L. M.: Validity of criterion measures for occupational therapists. Am J. Occup. Ther. 30:229, 1976.
2. Campbell, D. T., and Stanley, J. C.: Experimental and Quasi-experimental Designs for Research. Rand-McNally, Chicago, 1963.
3. Buros, O. K.: Mental Measurements Yearbook. Gryphon Press, Highland Park, N.J., 1972.

ADDITIONAL READING

Ethridge, D. A., and McSweeney, M.: Research in occupational therapy, part IV: Data collection and analysis. Am. J. Occup. Ther. 25:90, 1971.

Chapter 10

THE LIBRARY AS A TOOL

OBJECTIVES

1. *Discuss the role of the library search in research.*
2. *List the major resources in a typical medical library which can serve as entry points into the literature; state the major characteristics of each resource.*
3. *Give examples of how one can use the library to search for information on a given topic.*

THE LIBRARY SEARCH

The library serves several functions in the basic and continuing education of any professional. This chapter concerns the library as a research tool.

The purpose of reviewing the literature in a given field was mentioned in Chapter 1. Once you have identified your goal or established a research hypothesis, the review of related literature should answer two main questions: (1) Has my research question already been answered? (2) What have other people learned which will help me to answer my question?

The researcher should have at least a general goal in mind before he begins his library search. If he enters the library with only a general goal, he can read to get an overview of the entire area of interest. The library search will require three basic supplies: paper, pencils, and patience. It takes a long time to find, read, understand, and integrate information contained in the literature. Say, as an example, that you begin with the topic of human movement, or kinesiology. With an interest this large you would probably go to general textbooks on the subject in order to get a wide sampling of what is known in the area. Table 10-1 is an outline for reading in the subject of kinesiology; it gives an idea of the various directions which your research could explore. The student could spend considerable time getting just a superficial knowledge of what is known in each of the five major areas listed there.

Usually the researcher has already completed this initial mastery of the subject matter long before he approaches a specific research project. Such broad areas of interest are generally encompassed in an introductory course. What about the two therapists from St. Hopeless Hospital who were introduced in Chapter 1? Their original goal was improving joint mobility in patients with physical disabilities. They eventually decided to conduct a series of experiments with two specific goals in mind: (1) To evaluate the accuracy of various tools for measuring joint mobility, and (2) To evaluate several therapeutic procedures for increasing joint mobility. They developed a series of questions which we have examined throughout this textbook.

Before they could carry out any of those research projects, they had to review the related literature. If these therapists started with the outline in Table 10-1, their first goal would come under item III, Biomechanics. They could then outline their reading in this area as shown in Table 10-2. Much of this reading would still be at the secondary source (textbook) level of reading. Eventually, in order to address their first purpose of evaluating tools for measuring joint mobility,

Table 10-1. Outline for reading in the broad area of kinesiology

---
Goal: to understand how people achieve purposeful movement

   I. Structural and functional kinesiology
      A. Gross anatomy
      B. Functional anatomy
   II. Exercise physiology
 III. Biomechanics
 IV. Developmental studies
      A. Physiological
         1. Motor
         2. Sensory
      B. Psychosocial
   V. Psychological aspects of movement

Table 10-2. Outline for reading in biomechanics*

Biomechanics
  A. Statics
  B. Dynamics
    1. Kinetics
    2. Kinematics
      a. Planes of movement
      b. Levers and axes
        1) Types
        2) Measurement
      c. Displacement
      d. Normal ranges

*Heading III from Table 10-1.

they will get some very specific reading about measurement. They are then ready to read seriously in the primary sources to get an in-depth understanding of what has been done and what is known about the measurement of joint mobility. They have completed the first three steps in writing a research protocol (Appendix A).

As the researchers approach their task they should always keep their specific research questions in mind so that they do not get distracted by interesting, irrelevant reading. What methodology and procedures did other workers in the same area use? The reading may suggest new ideas and techniques which had not originally occurred to them.

As they read they will take careful notes. Many researchers use index cards for this purpose. At the top of the card there might be a notation which would refer to a heading from an outline such as those found in Tables 10-1 and 10-2 which would quickly identify the main topic covered by the card. Full bibliographic references should be written down clearly with attention to spelling and page numbers so that the researcher does not have to go back to the literature later when he is compiling references. A full bibliographic reference includes the author's full name, the title of the article, the journal or book title, volume, page numbers, and year of publication. For books, the publisher and city of publication and the edition are necessary.

The researcher should then take careful notes of all information which is relevant to the research question, as well as anything that is related to the broader topic of joint mobility. At the bottom or on the back of the card it is helpful to make a few brief notes about how the article relates to your question and how you think you might be able to use the information in developing your research protocol.

Look over the hypotheses in Chapter 1; it is obvious that the therapists from St. Hopeless are going to need information about standard goniometry and electrogoniometry since both measuring devices are involved in several of their hypotheses. The next question they must answer, then, is: How can the relevant primary literature be located in that mass of material in the medical library?

ENTRY POINTS INTO THE LITERATURE

You step through the front door of the library and there they are: several floors, jam-packed with thousands of books and bound journals. Where do you begin? There are a number of reference resources which are organized for the express purpose of assisting you in your review of the literature. But even with all of these aids, the beginning researcher should be reminded that one of the major requirements of an effective library searching is patience. Be organized and take good notes to avoid the frustration of repeated searching.

The major entry points into a medical library are as follows:

Card catalogues
Computer
Index Medicus
Reference books
  Books in Print
  Annual reviews
  Journal indices
  Excerpta Medica and other abstract compilations
Citation index
The librarian

Let's take a brief look at each one of these.

Card Catalogues

The card catalogues are the heart of the library and the most important single entry point into everything in the library's holdings. There is at least one card for every piece of literature in the library, including books, journals (but not individual journal articles), filmstrips, microfilm, microfiche, audio, and video tapes. In most libraries there are three separate sets of cards, one for authors, one for subjects, and one for titles. Each is arranged in alphabetical order. It is assumed that the reader is already familiar with the general layout of libraries and the card catalogues, so a great deal of time will not be spent on this. If any reader is not familiar with the card catalogues and the call numbers (either Library of Congress system or the Dewey decimal system), he should ask for assistance from one of the general librarians.

The researcher who is at the general goal level in his project (Tables 10-1 and 10-2) will find the subject heading catalogue most useful. When you have identified an interesting looking title in the card catalogue, go to the shelves to find that book. Look also at other books on the same shelf, and other books with the same general number. For example, Brunnstrom's *Clinical Kinesiology* has the Library of Congress number QP301. Other books with the same number will be in the same general subject area and can often provide you with a whole shelf full of references. The references and bibliographies in the books you have located will alert you to other secondary sources and many primary sources upon which textbook material is based. When you write down a reference which you find in a textbook such as Brunnstrom, it is helpful also to note where you found the reference in case you make some mistake in transcribing and need to go back to your source. If Brunnstrom refers to a textbook by Wells, you can go back to the author headings in the card catalogue to find that book if you have not already discovered it on the same shelf with Brunnstrom.

In order to illustrate some of the complexities of the card catalogues, the author searched for the Brunnstrom book in the subject card catalogue. It was not under kinesiology; in fact, there was no subject heading for kinesiology in the cards. It was not found under anatomy or functional anatomy either. Brunnstrom was finally found under the subject heading "movement." When searching in card catalogues, with the computer, or in references such as *Index Medicus*, an awareness of synonyms can prove most helpful.

Computers

The computer provides an entry point into recent literature which is not confined to a single library. It can often reduce the amount of time spent in library search by as much as one half. In order to use the computer in your search you need two things: a key word or a set of key words which will be recognized by the computer, and a reference librarian.

There are two major computer systems which should be of interest to readers of this book, one is called MEDLARS and the other ERIC. MEDLARS stands for "Medical Literature Analysis and Retrieval System"; this is maintained by the National Library of Medicine and contains several hundred million references. All of the references in MEDLARS are filed under the key words used by *Index Medicus*.

(This key to *Index Medicus* is explained in detail later.) Therefore, in order to get into the computer data base in MEDLARS you must know certain key phrases. The reference librarian can be of assistance to you in learning to understand computer language. ERIC stands for "Education Resources Information Center," and is a computerized data base maintained by the U.S. Office of Education. Another computer data base of interest is called Psychological Abstracts and is maintained by the American Psychological Association. Both ERIC and Psychological Abstracts have lists of key words.

Frequently the reference librarian is able to obtain an immediate print-out of 20 or so of the most recent items; this is called "on-line" service. It may be possible to get several pages of print-out. If you want an exhaustive search that goes all the way back to the beginning of the computerized data base, you may have to wait a week or more.

If you are interested in a topic such as goniometry, which does not appear in the indexing keys, you can "ask" the computer to give you a print-out of all articles which have that word in their title. This approach is ordinarily used when you don't know any other way of gaining access to the material. With the assistance of a reference librarian the author asked MEDLARS to search on-line for articles with the word goniometry in the title. Covering only the last three years, an immediate print-out of four articles resulted, after which the computer typed "end of documents and list—enter return or another command," meaning, those are the only four articles with the word goniometry in the title submitted to the MEDLARS data base over the last three years. The first reference on the computer print-out looks like this:

AU Townsend, M.A., Izak, M. and Jackson, R.W.
 TI Total Motion Knee Goniometry
SO J Biomech. 10:3:183–193, 1977
MJ Knee
MN Adult, Aged, Arthritis, Biomechanics, Gait, Human, Male, Movement

This computer print-out may be translated as follows: the authors of the first article are Townsend, Isak, and Jackson. The article title is *Total Motion Knee Goniometry*; it appeared in the *Journal of Biomechanics*, volume 10, number 3, pages 183 to 193, in 1977. MJ stands for major keys; this article's major computer listing is "knee." The last line lists minor keys under which it is also listed; note that this particular article can be found by the computer under any of eight minor key words. This list of key words might give the researcher some cues as to other ways to approach the computer's data base.

130

Index Medicus

Before the advent of MEDLARS (which is a kind of computerized *Index Medicus*), the *Index Medicus* was the major entry point into periodical medical literature. The *Index Medicus* is published on a monthly basis and bound into a multi-volume set by years. The yearly edition lists all journals which are indexed in the *Index Medicus*; both *Physical Therapy* and the *American Journal of Occupational Therapy* are among the journals indexed. The January issue includes a list entitled "Medical Subject Headings." These are the key phrases used in the MEDLARS data base as well as the topic headings under which journal articles appear in the *Index Medicus*. In the early part of a search the reader may find it helpful to go to the list of medical subject headings to find the keys under which his topic may be found.

In looking for the literature on goniometry while preparing some of the examples and illustrations used in this text, the author discovered that the word goniometry is not in the list of medical subject headings. The words test and measurements are also not usable keys. After some searching around in the list of headings, the author found "Physical Examination." Under this major heading there are four subheadings: instrumentation, methods, standards, and veterinary. In the cumulated *Index Medicus* for 1976 under the topic heading "Physical Examination," subheading "instrumentation," three articles are listed. One of these articles was published in 1974, another in 1975, and another in 1976; this points to the fact that articles don't always get into the *Index Medicus* the year they are published. Two of these three articles are concerned with goniometry. One was published in the *Medical Journal of Zambia* and the other in *Plastic and Reconstructive Surgery*. Under "methods" 17 articles are listed. Five of these are in foreign languages (the language is specified). Of those 17 articles one is clearly related to goniometry because the word hydrogoniometer appears in the title. Another article, "Measurement of Spinal Mobility: A Comparison of Three Methods," may deal with goniometry but you would have to check the original article to be sure. None of the seven articles under the key subheading "standards" dealt with goniometry.

With this information the serious searcher now has two choices. He can go through every year of the *Index Medicus*, beginning with the latest and working backward, and check under the subheadings, "instrumentation" and "methods" under "Physical Examination." Or if the computer is available, one could ask the computer to print out everything listed under "Physical Examination: Instrumentation and Methods." It might also be wise to include the subsection "standards," since on the basis of one year only it cannot be totally ruled out as a key to literature of interest.

Reference Books

Other entry points into the literature, when you have only a general topic to search, are reference books. There are many useful reference books and not all of them can be listed here. There are, however, a few important ones which are likely to be of interest to readers of this book.

Books in Print

Books in Print comprises three huge volumes; one for authors, one for subjects, one for titles. These list all of the books currently available from publishers in the United States. There is also a *British Books in Print.* These are most useful when you have a broad topic to search or if you have discovered an author whose books you like and want to know what else he has written. The subject guide of *Books in Print* has a section on kinesiology.

Annual Reviews

There is also a series of books published under the general title of *"Annual Review of _____."* Two examples are *Annual Review of Physiology* and *Annual Review of Psychology.* Typically each chapter in these reviews is written by a different expert who reviews the latest information and thinking on a given topic. Not every topic is covered every year. For example, in the *Annual Review of Psychology*, the topic of human performance is reviewed only every fourth year. These review articles are also listed separately in the *Index Medicus.*

Journal Indices

Many journals print an index in the December issue of the journal. Articles are usually indexed by both author and title, and sometimes also by general subject heading. Also, some journals—*Physical Therapy* and the *American Journal of Occupational Therapy* among them—publish cumulative indices every 5, 25, or 50 years. These indices are helpful in obtaining the entire history of developments in a particular area.

There are a number of journals or books which print nothing but abstracts of articles which appear in journals. An abstract includes a bibliographic reference and a brief summary of what the article had to say. Four important publications in this area are: *Psychological Abstracts, Biological Abstracts, Dissertation Abstracts* and *Excerpta Medica. Excerpta Medica* is especially useful since its several yearly volumes cover a variety of disciplines, i.e., anatomy, pediatrics, neurology, geriatrics, internal medicine, rehabilitation. Abstracts in *Excerpta Medica* are taken from journals published all over the world; they are not necessarily the same journals in *Index Medicus*, although there is a large overlap. *Excerpta Medica* publishes over 40 sections a year. Section XIX is "Rehabilitation and Physical Medicine." Each recent volume on rehabilitation is divided into 20 subtopics and many of these have subsections of their own. These include sections on functional tests, physical therapy, occupational therapy, and activities of daily living.

In looking for literature on goniometry the author went to *Excerpta Medica*, section XIX, "Rehabilitation and Physical Medicine," Volume 20, 1977. Under subsection 6.0, "Functional Tests," there were three abstracts of articles dealing with goniometry by three different authors: Low, Bojd and Owen. Abstract 1248 gave the following bibliographic reference.

AU Low, JL (Auckland)
TI The Reliability of Joint Measurement
SO *Physiotherapy.* 62:7:227–229, 1976

That article was then abstracted in two short paragraphs so that the reader would know whether or not he wanted to read the entire article. In the same volume there is also an author index and a cumulative subject index. Under the cumulative subject index there is a subject heading "Goniometry," that lists the abstracts of Low and Bojd which had been found in the main body of the volume as well as two others; both of these dealt primarily with knee evaluation and therefore had not been listed under functional tests. The author then found the subject heading "Electrogoniometry," that included the article by Owen which had been found under "Functional Tests," as well as three other articles which did not deal primarily with functional tests but made some mention of electrogoniometry. One of these latter three was an article which appeared in Volume 30 of the *American Journal of Occupational Therapy.*

In *Excerpta Medica*, Section XIX, Volume 13, 1970, the author found the subject heading index "Electrogoniometry," under which abstract 967 was listed. Going into the main body of the volume, abstract 967 gave the following reference:

AU Johnston, RC and GL Smidt
TI "Measurement of Hip Joint Motion during Walking: Evaluation of an Electrogoniometric Method"
SO J. Bone and Jt. Surg. (Boston) 51A:6:1083–1094, 1969.

This is one of the references which will be used in Table 11–3 in the next chapter. This reference will also be used later in this chapter to illustrate the uses of the *Citation Index*.

Citation Index

The fifth resource listed earlier is the *Citation Index*. There are two branches of the *Citation Index*: the *Science Citation Index* and the *Social Science Citation Index*.

The *Science Citation Index* is published quarterly; cumulations are published yearly and every five years. It has four sections: the Citation Index, the Source Index, the Permuterm Subject Index, and the Corporate Index. These are most useful after you have found an article which is in some way important to your research question. Unfortunately, neither *Physical Therapy* nor the *American Journal of Occupational Therapy* are indexed by *Citation Index*. However, it is still useful for articles found in other journals. Having found the reference in *Excerpta Medica* to the article by Johnston and Smidt the author went to the five-year cumulative index of *Science Citation Index* for the years 1970 through 1974. The original article had been published in 1969. In the Citation Index section the author found the article by Johnston and Smidt listed. Under it were 19 articles which *referred to* the Johnston article in their reviews of related literature. The seventh article listed was the following:

J. Bone JT. Surg. A52:775, 1970, Kettelka.

Following the citation to the article by Kettelka in the *Journal of Bone and Joint Surgery*, the author went to the Source Index section of the *Science Citation Index* and looked up Kettelka in the cumulative five-year index for 1970–74. There was a long list of articles published by him during that five-year period, including the 1970 article in the *Journal of Bone and Joint Surgery*. Kettelka was senior author, the other authors were Johnson, Smidt, et al. The full title of the article is "An Electrogoniometric Study of Knee Motion in Normal Gait." It

134

wasn't until the author went to the bound volumes of the *Journal of Bone and Joint Surgery* and found the article itself that he discovered that Kettelka is an abbreviated form for "Kettelkamp."

The third section of the *Science Citation Index* is the Permuterm Subject Index. Looking in the five-year cumulation from 1970 to 1974 under the subject heading, "Electrogoniometric," there was only one article listed—the one by Kettelka. Continuing in the Permuterm Subject Index, under "Goniometer" there were approximately 300 articles listed. Each one is identified with a key term so that for each article you have a pair of terms, such as goniometer-account, goniometer-device, goniometer-electronic, goniometer–x-ray, etc. There were also approximately 50 articles under the term "Goniometers," another 100 under "Goniometric," and 9 under "Goniometry." There were about 12 articles listed under "Gonio-photography."

The Librarian

The last general entry point into the literature which was listed earlier in this chapter is the librarian. She is last, but certainly not least. The librarian is listed last only with the idea in mind that the researcher should make some attempt to solve his own problems before going to the librarian.

Table 10–3. Guide to a library search

If you have a topic—
    Card catalog, subject index
    Computer
        MEDLARS
        ERIC
        Psychological Abstracts
    Index Medicus
        Medical Subject Headings
    Reference books
        Books in Print, subject index
        Annual reviews
        Journal indices
        Abstracts, especially *Excerpta Medica*, subject index
    Citation Index
        Permuterm Subject Index
If you have a name (author)—
    Card catalog, author index
    Computer, author entry
    Index Medicus, author index
    Reference books, author indices
    Citation Index
        Citation index
        Source index
If you have a reference—
    Bibliography
    Citation Index

GUIDE TO LIBRARY SEARCH

Table 10-3 is a generalized guide to a library search for purposes of research. If you have only a general topic, there are a number of places to go to get into the literature: subject headings in the card catalogues or the *Index Medicus* or the computer data base, various reference books, and the Permuterm Subject Index of the *Citation Index*. If you have the name of a well-known author in your area of interest, you can look under the various author listings. Finally, if you have a good primary source which is relevant to your research question, you can follow it in two directions: backwards, by looking at the references cited by the author in *his* review of literature; and forward, through the *Citation Index* list of articles which mention it in *their* reviews of the literature.

REVIEW QUESTIONS

1. Return to review question 1 in Chapter 9 and answer it again using the new information you have acquired in this chapter.
2. Start with a general research goal in an area of interest. Use the library to do a superficial review and make note of particularly helpful resources. Narrow the area down to a more specific research purpose and research it. Finally, write a research hypothesis and do a thorough review of the relevant literature using the guide provided in Table 10-3.

ADDITIONAL READING

Lehmkuhl, D.: Techniques for locating, filing and retrieving scientific information. Phys. Ther. 58:579, 1978.

Chapter 11

THEORY REVISITED

OBJECTIVE

1. *Based on the models presented in the text, outline a general model which might be used to guide research in your discipline.*

THE USES OF THEORY

It might be a good idea at this point to reread Chapter 2 in the light of everything else that has been learned in this textbook. In Chapter 2 we defined theory as a set of principles which are based on solid evidence and which organize what is known about a subject in a way which is useful for generating new principles. In expanding on that definition, an emphasis was placed on solid evidence, organization, and utilization. In the introduction and in Chapter 1 the role of research in the validation of clinical practice was discussed.

In all professions, and most especially in new and developing professions such as physical and occupational therapy, there is a continuous and urgent need to substantiate and further solidify the principles upon which clinical practice is built. There is an equally pressing need to organize those principles so that they assist the clinician in developing new principles which will improve practice. In other words, there is an urgent need for occupational and physical therapists to make explicit the theories on which they are now operating, and to develop those theories so that they can act as a stimulus to further development. Of particular importance in this context is the idea that important, researchable questions will be highlighted in the process of writing out the theories on which we operate, and in the process of operationally defining terms and organizing what is known into a theory format (see Chapter 2). By this process of theory building it will become much more obvious what information is missing, so that wasted effort can be avoided and high priority questions can be identified more quickly.

BASIC VERSUS APPLIED RESEARCH

The model by Hilgard and Bower[1] was mentioned in Chapter 7 in the discussion of educational research. This model is shown in Table 11-1, and has been modified in Table 11-2 to make it relevant to clinical practice. It is proposed as a model which can be used in conjunction with the model of a theory proposed in Chapter 2, the protocol guide in Appendix A, the guide to library research in Chapter 10 (Table 10-3), and the measurement guide which is presented in this chapter (Table 11-3). These five form a combination of tools which may be used to validate and expand clinical practice. They are certainly not the only tools available, and like any other tools they should be used only when their use is productive and disregarded in other instances.

The original model outlined by Hilgard and Bower listed three steps under basic science research and three steps under technological research and development in the field of education. Table 11-1 outlines the Hilgard-Bower model and gives one example of each step. A similar model was developed by Smidt[2]; his six steps were (1) fundamental, (2) design and development, (3) evaluation and standardization on normals, (4) evaluation and standardization on abnormals, (5) clinical application, and (6) clinical implementation. Smidt's system is

Table 11-1. The Hilgard–Bowers research model

Basic Science Research
    Step 1. Not directly relevant to education, e.g., animal maze learning
    Step 2. Topic-relevant, e.g., concept learning
    Step 3. School-relevant, e.g., learning math concepts

Technological Research and Development
    Step 4. School laboratory research, e.g., studies using special settings and special teachers
    Step 5. Normal classroom "try-out," e.g., step 4 repeated in normal setting
    Step 6. Adoption, e.g., write textbooks and train teachers to use step 4 process or materials.

Table 11-2. A generalized model for research in occupational and physical therapy

BASIC

Step 1. Microbiological Research
  A. Elasticity of tendon *in vivo*
  B. Movement time in manual dexterity
  C. Nonphysical affective stimulation in children ages 6 to 12
Step 2. Biological Systems Research
  A. Mechanisms of diarthroidial articulation
  B. Eye-hand coordination in manual tasks
  C. Normal affect related to body image in children ages 6 to 12
Step 3. Pathokinesiology
  A. Typical course of rheumatoid arthritis in the knee joint—histological and mechanical
  B. Measurement of manual dexterity in spastic victims of cerebral palsy
  C. Body image in children ages 6 to 12 with congenital spasticity in comparison to children with acquired spasticity

APPLIED

Step 4. Therapeutic Kinesiology
  A. Influence of active exercise on range of motion in rheumatoid knees
  B. Influence of rhythmic stabilization exercises for shoulder, elbow, and wrist on subsequent hand dexterity in patients with spastic cerebral palsy
  C. Influence of group socialization activities on body image of spastic children ages 6 to 12
Step 5. Therapeutic Regimens
  A. Interactive effects of drugs, exercise, and heat modalities on function of rheumatoid knees
  B. Interactive effects of drugs, exercise, and vocational training on employment of spastic adults in light industry
  C. Interactive effects of group socialization activities, rational-emotive therapy, and ADL training on spastic children ages 6 to 12

particularly well suited to the development and evaluation of clinical and research instruments and therapeutic modalities.

GENERALIZED RESEARCH MODEL (TABLE 11-2)

Table 11-2 is a model for research relevant to occupational and physical therapy. It was developed for this text using Hilgard and Smidt as guides. In the context of this model, kinesiology is defined as a study of human movement which encompasses all aspects of and influences on movement—biological, psychological, and social. The model has five steps. The first three are classified as basic research and the last two are classified as applied research. Under each step three examples are given. In each instance, example A is in the physical-biological area, example B is in the psychomotor area, and example C is in the psychosocial area. These examples are not intended to be specific research hypotheses or even goals or purposes. They are

general areas of interest. All five A examples are loosely intercon-
nected, as are the B examples and C examples, but no clear-cut progression is intended through the five steps at any of the levels; it is,
then, only a generalized model.

Let us first examine the five basic steps. Step 1 is Microbiological
Research. It is "micro" because it looks at only one small part of a
larger phenomenon; it is biological in the sense that it refers to life, and
in this case, to human life. Example A is at the tissue level, example B
deals with only one small component of the concept of manual dexterity and example C is looking for a general list of non-physical things
that stimulate affective responses in children.

Step 2 is Biological Systems Research. Example A is concerned with
the general mechanisms of all kinds of dyarthroidal articulations. Example B deals with one aspect of the complex required to perform a
manual task. Example C is concerned with normal children and one affective attitude, that of body image.

In a sense, step 3 is at the same level of step 2 in that it is looking at
biological systems. But step 3 is looking at biological systems which
have pathology present. In another sense, there is a sequence between
steps 2 and 3 since the student usually finds it helpful to understand
normal before trying to define the pathological. The examples follow
the same sequence of biological, motor, and psychosocial.

Research done in steps 1 and 2 is frequently done by anatomists,
physiologists. psychologists, and sociologists. Research at these two
levels is done by occupational and physical therapists with advanced
training in the basic sciences. However, it could also be done by people
with no knowledge or interest in these therapeutic professions. Step 3
deals with subject matter of particular interest to therapists and
research at step 3 can and should be done in research laboratories
staffed, at least in part, by physical and occupational therapists. In
working out the details of many questions in this area, and in interpreting the data generated at step 3, the therapist would frequently
call upon the expertise of basic scientists and medical specialists to
contribute to the development of principles in pathokinesiology.

In steps 4 and 5 we have moved into the applied sphere, clinical
therapeutics. The examples in step 4 deal with therapeutic elements in
a laboratory setting. The kinds of questions which would be asked in
step 4 tend to isolate one independent variable at a time and study its
effects on selected measurements. Step 4, which would encompass
nonmovement modalities that facilitate or inhibit movement as well
as movement modalities, relates fairly closely to Hilgard's step 4:
laboratory research using special settings and specially trained clinicians. Step 4 is designated as applied research because active exercise

usually is not the only treatment for rheumatoid knees (example A), and rhythmic stabilization usually is not the only therapeutic technique used in training spastic victims of cerebral palsy (example B). The major purpose in step 4 is to isolate independent variables and to identify their specific effects. Research at this level is almost always the exclusive domain of therapists.

As Hilgard's step 5 was normal classroom research, so step 5 in this model is normal clinical research. It represents an attempt to define the cumulative effect of a total therapeutic regimen. If the health care team gives its best to patients with rheumatoid knees, a number of therapeutic modalities will most likely be applied under the supervision of physicians, nurses, physical therapists, and occupational therapists. These various aspects of treatment interact with one another. Drug therapy enhances or inhibits the effectiveness of exercise procedures. Conversely, the effects of exercise may support or oppose the action of certain drugs. Our ultimate concern is the total welfare of the patient and therefore the ultimate research questions must be the total net effect of the entire therapeutic complex on the life and well-being of one human being. That one individual is often studied as a member of a group of similar human beings, but the therapist should never lose sight of the most important question of all: What good are we doing this person, and how are we doing it? Step 5 of our model looks at the therapeutic environment and asks questions about the net effect of that total environment on individuals or groups. Therapists can do this kind of research singly, as primary investigators with proper input from the other health professionals involved in the care of the patients, or they can do it as members of an interdisciplinary team of researchers.

USES OF THE RESEARCH MODEL

This generalized model serves several useful purposes. To the reader it may serve as a reminder to evaluate each bit of newly acquired information, and determine where it can best contribute to the overall understanding of the problem. Earlier in this text we discussed the danger of taking results from animal research and applying them clinically without researching the appropriateness of that application. Many clinicians have been unnecessarily disillusioned and disheartened by failing to see the necessary progression, and by assuming that an answer to a question at step 1 is equivalent to the answer to a question which should be asked at step 4 or step 5 of the model in Table 11–2.

The second use of the model is to assist the student in organizing what he knows about a given topic and in developing a set of definitions, postulates, and hypotheses about a given topic. If the definitions and postulates are at step 1, are the hypotheses at step 2 or do they jump to step 5? For example, Tokizane[3] published a study in which, among other things, he studied the labyrinthine reflex and its influence on flexor and extensor muscle tone. His subjects were five normal adults and one adult deaf-mute. He concluded that with the head in a specific position, stimulation of the labyrinthine reflex would facilitate extensor tone and decrease flexor tone in selected muscles throughout the body. On the basis of that information, would you put a brain-damaged child or adult in a head-down, inverted position to stimulate the extensor tone in their musculature? What about the influence of that position on other reflexes or its influence on systems other than the muscular? What is its influence on the cardiovascular system? What neurological mechanisms may be stimulated or inhibited by this method of stimulating the labyrinthine reflex? All of those questions are still in steps 1 and 2, as was Tokizane's research. What about the myriad of questions that need to be answered in step 3? What does the presence of various kinds of pathology do to influence the labyrinthine reflex and all of its neuromuscular connections? What are the specific therapeutic effects of the inverted position in different types of patients and in individual patients, and, finally, what are the interactive effects of the inverted position with other therapeutic procedures which may be applied to patients with cerebral palsy or hemiplegia?

A third potential use of the model grows out of the second one; the model may suggest specific questions which need answering and a general approach to answering them. Suppose that a clinician learns of a new therapeutic modality and wants to answer some questions about its effectiveness on his patients. The question of interest is clearly at step 4 or step 5. The model suggests that there are some more basic questions underlying the question of clinical interest. A search of the literature may provide some of these answers and information from the earlier stages can assist the clinician in refining the question in ways that will make his research project as useful as possible.

What has been said so far is not intended to imply that research *must* progress from step 1 through step 5. In some instances that may be the ideal progression and it is certainly the most efficient approach for long-term studies. However, there are times when this progression is not feasible and there are probably times when it is not the most fruitful. Therapeutic procedures which have grown out of clinical experience and empirical trial and error may generate defendable hypotheses at the clinical level. People with a basic science interest and expertise may then take these clinically demonstrable facts, develop hypotheses that will explain the underlying mechanisms at steps 1, 2, and 3, and thus support the clinical practice in question. In an earlier chapter the example was given of the development of smallpox vaccine which was clinically effective before the microbiological basis of the disease and of the vaccine was discovered. The essential point here is that the model is not a magic formula; it is a tool to be used creatively in the search for more reliable knowledge.

A separate step, dissemination of information, was not included in the model because it is a component of each of the five steps. The researcher has a clear obligation to report the results of his studies so that his professional colleagues can share the information and use it. Publishing results is thus a professional obligation as much as it is a specific step in the research process. Dissemination of information is also most relevant to education and professional development.

MEASUREMENT EVALUATION MODEL

The purpose of this textbook has been to provide the reader with knowledge and skills which facilitate his intellectual defense of therapeutic procedures. This knowledge and these skills are prerequisites to the development of new knowledge through research. To assist the reader in these tasks, the text has provided a number of concepts and principles which help to explain the research process. In addition, four models have been provided as guides to assist the serious reader in organizing knowledge and thoughts relative to clinical practice. These four models, mentioned earlier, are (1) the model for the development of a theory presented in Chapter 2, (2) the model for a research protocol located in Appendix B, (3) the guide for a literature search presented in Chapter 10, and (4) the generalized model for research in physical and occupational therapy discussed earlier in this chapter. A fifth model, a guide for evaluating measurement tools, is presented below.

Evaluating Measurement Tools

In Chapter 4 we suggested that as research becomes more precise it tends to move from nominal to metric levels of measurement. This is only a tendency and is not always necessarily so, but it is usually a desirable trend. The selection of the dependent measure is not always a quick and clear-cut decision. Frequently, there are a number of available measurement tools for the same dependent variable. The researcher must make decisions which often involve selecting a tool

143

that is particularly strong in one desirable component but weak in another. Table 11-3 is a guide to assist the researcher in evaluating available measurement tools and reaching a decision about which one is appropriate for a particular study. A modified version of this guide was presented at a 1973 graduate education workshop.[4] In Table 11-3 goniometry has been chosen as the dependent measure to be used as an example so that this model can be related more easily to other models developed in the text.

The left-hand column lists measurement tools or instruments which may be used to measure the dependent variable, identified at the top of the table. Each instrument is then evaluated on the basis of six criteria. The first criterion is that of relevance, and answers the question: To what extent does the measurement tool measure an important aspect of the research question? The second criterion is that of validity: To what extent does the instrument sample the attributes of the independent variable that it is supposed to measure? The third criterion is that of power: To what extent does the tool differentiate among things that are different? The fourth criterion is reliability: How ac-

Table 11-3. A guide for evaluating measurement tools*

Dependent Variable: Goniometry

Rank each measure 1 (highest) to 5 (lowest).

Measures or Instruments	Measures an important aspect of question (relevance)	Samples the attributes it is supposed to measure (validity)	Differentiates among things that are different (power)	Accurately reflects changes in performance (reliability)	Communicates results in unambiguous terms (interpretable)	Value of measure is worth the cost of data collection (feasibility)
1. Subjective assessment[1,4]	2	4	5	5	5	2
2. Protractor goniometer[1,3,5,7]	1	1	2	2[8]	1	1
3. Photographic[2]	1	1	2	3	1	3
4. Pendulum arthrometer[1,7]	1	1	2	3	1	1
5. Special use goniometers[7]						
a. Pronation-supination[7]	1	1	2	2[8]	1	1
b. Fingers[6,7,10]	1	1	2	3[9]	1	1
c. Ankle[11]	1	1	2	2[11]	1	1
d. Hip[15]	1	1[15]	1	2[15]	1	2
6. Electrogoniometer[12,13,14,15]	1[14]	1[12,13]	1[12,13]	2[12,13]	1[13,14]	2

*Note: References cited are listed at the end of this chapter in a separate listing.

curately does the instrument reflect changes in performance or performance variability as opposed to error variability? The fifth criterion is that of interpretability: To what extent do the measurement data effectively communicate results in unambiguous terms? The last criterion is that of feasibility: Given the evaluation of the tool with regard to the other five criteria, is it worth the cost in time and money?

The value of this approach will vary with different dependent variables. In our example of goniometry, there is little difference in the power of the several instruments. However, if we were dealing with psychological measures or measures of perceptual motor performance, there would be a much wider variability among instruments on each of the criteria of evaluation. The guide is useful for developing the various research designs discussed in Chapters 5 through 8. This is probably least obvious in descriptive research of the questionnaire/survey type; however, even there some of the criteria can be applied to individual questions in the questionnaire. Is the question phrased in such a way that it truly samples the attributes we wish to measure by this question? Does it differentiate people who are basically different in the attributes that we are trying to measure? Is it clear and unambiguous?

A detailed knowledge of and familiarity with the measurement instruments available is required in order to fully utilize this guide. Therefore, its use will usually involve some library research. For clarity, accuracy, and preservation of information it is helpful to reference, wherever possible, the decisions that are made about each instrument. Therefore, Table 11-3 includes references to the information on which some of the ranking decisions were made.

SUMMARY

The diligent reader should now have the basic tools for reading, understanding and using the evidence provided by their professional literature. Like any other skill, from algebraic equations to piano playing, skill in reading and interpreting research comes with practice, and one can frequently learn as much from mistakes as from success. Once some modicum of skill is developed in reading, interpreting, and applying other people's research, and in understanding how they arrived at their results, conclusions, and interpretations, the reader is then ready to embark, at some modest and meaningful level, on the high and rewarding adventure of making an original contribution to our understanding of useful therapeutic procedures.

REVIEW QUESTIONS

As a final self-examination the reader is invited to attempt the following procedures:

1. Select a topic of interest about which you have some interest.
2. Do a review of the literature concerning what is known about that topic. Use the guide developed in Chapter 10 and analyze each reading critically, following the outline suggested in Appendix A.
3. Organize what you have learned in the form of a formal statement of the theory underlying the therapeutic procedure which you are studying. Use the model of a theory developed in Chapter 2 for this purpose.
4. Spread out the information which you gathered in steps 2 and 3 above using the research model developed in the first half of this chapter. In which of the five steps in Table 11-2 are most of your concepts and principles located?
5. Identify several research questions which you believe to be important and useful.
6. Select the research question which you believe you are most capable of answering and most willing to devote time and energy to. Develop that question into a research protocol using the model provided in Appendix A. When selecting your dependent variable, use the model for evaluating dependent measures presented in Table 11-3.
7. Execute the study. (Remember, where there's a will, there's a way—and enjoy!)

REFERENCES

1. Hilgard, E. R., and Bower, G. H.: Theories of Learning, ed. 3. Appleton-Century-Crofts, New York, 1966.
2. Smidt, G.: Research in musculo-skeletal disorders. Paper presented to the Section on Research, American Physical Therapy Association, Houston, Texas, June 27, 1973.
3. Tokizane, T., et al.: Electromyographic studies on tonic neck, lumbar and labyrinthine reflexes in normal persons. Jpn. J. Physiol. 2:130, 1951.
4. American Physical Therapy Association: Teaching Objective Measurement in Graduate Physical Therapy Education. Unpublished proceedings of a workshop sponsored by the Graduate Education Committee, Ashville, N.C., 1973.

REFERENCES FOR TABLE 11-3

1. Salter, N.: Methods of measurement of muscle and joint function. J. Bone Joint Surg. 37B(3)474, 1955.
2. Wilson, G. D., and Stasch, W. H.: Photographic record of joint motion. Arch. Phys Med. Rehabil. 26:361, 1945.

3. Zankel, H. T.: Photogoniometry. Arch. Phys. Med. Rehabil. 32:277, 1951.
4. Zimmerman, M. E.: The functional motion test as an evaluation tool for patients with lower motor neuron disturbances. Am. J. Occup. Ther. 23:49, 1969.
5. Hurt, S. P.: Joint measurement. Am. J. Occup. Ther. 1(4):209; 1(5):281; 2(1):13, 1947.
6. Devore, G., and Smith, H.: A new method for measuring motion of flexor tendon grafts. Am. J. Occup. Ther. 24(5):336, 1970.
7. Moore, M. L.: The measurement of joint motion, part I: Introduction and review of the literature. Phys. Ther. 29:195. 1949.
8. Hellebrandt, F. A., et al.: The measurement of joint motion. Part III: Reliability of goniometry. Phys. Ther. 24:302, 1949.
9. Hamilton, G. F., and Lackenbruch, P. A.: Reliability of goniometers in assessing finger joint angle. Phys. Ther. 49:465, 1969.
10. Brayman, S.: Measuring device for joint motion of the hand. Am. J. Occup. Ther. 25:173, 1971.
11. Etter, M. F.: Measurement of motion at the ankle in the presence of deformity. Am. J. Occup. Ther. 18:244, 1964.
12. Karpovich, P. V., et al.: Electrogoniometric study of joints. USAF. Med. J. 11:424, 1966.
13. Finley, F. R., and Karpovich, P. V.: Electrogoniometric analysis of normal and pathological gaits. Res. Q. Am. Assoc. Health Phys. Educ. 35:379, 1964.
14. Tipton, C. M., and Karpovich, P. V.: Clinical electrogoniometry J.A.P.M.R. 2, Phys. Med. Rehab. 18(4):90, 1964.
15. Johnston, R. C., and Smidt, G. L.: Measurement of hip-joint motion during walking. J. Bone Joint Surg. 51A(6):1083, 1969.

BIBLIOGRAPHY FOR TEXT

Statistics (these are in order of difficulty—easy to hard)

Baggaley, A. R.: Mathematics for Introductory Statistics: A Programmed Review. John Wiley & Sons, N.Y., 1969.
McCollough, C., and Van Atta L.: Statistical Concepts: A Program for Self- Instruction. McGraw-Hill, N.Y., 1963.
Gilbert, N.: Statistics. W. B. Saunders, Philadelphia, 1976.
Sellers, G. R.: Elementary Statistics. W. B. Saunders, Philadelphia, 1977.
Kuebler, R. R., and Smith, H.: Statistics: A Beginning. John Wiley, N.Y., 1976.
Siegel, S.: Nonparametric Statistics for the Behavioral Sciences. McGraw-Hill, N.Y., 1956.
Huntsberger, D. V., and Leaverton, P. E.: Statistical Inference in the Biomedical Sciences. Allyn and Bacon, Boston, 1970.
Walker, H.: Elementary Statistical Methods. Rinehart and Winston, N.Y., 1943.
Colten, T.: Statistics in Medicine. Little, Brown, and Co., Boston, 1974.
Dotson, C. O., and Kirkendall, D. R.: Statistics for Physical Education, Health and Recreation. Harper and Row, N.Y., 1974.
Kilpatrick, S. J.: Statistical Principles in Health Care Information, ed. 2. University Park Press, Baltimore, 1977.
Kerlinger, F. N.: Foundations of Behavioral Research. Holt, Rinehart and Winston, N.Y., 1967.
Remington, R. D., and Schosk, M. A.: Statistics with Applications to the Biological and Health Sciences. Prentice-Hall, Englewood Cliffs, N.J., 1970.
Steele, R. G. D., and Torrie, H. H.: Principles and Procedures of Statistics. McGraw-Hill, N.Y., 1960.
Weinberg, G. M., and Schumaker, J. A.: Statistics: An Intuitive Approach, ed. 3. Brooks-Cole, Belmont, Cal., 1974.

Walker, H. M., and Lev, J.: Statistical Inference. Holt, Rinehart and Winston, N.Y., 1953.
Kirk, R. E.: Experimental Design: Procedures for the Behavioral Sciences. Brooks-Cole, Belmont, Cal., 1968.
Winer, B. J.: Statistical Principles in Experimental Design, ed. 2. McGraw-Hill, N.Y., 1971.

Writing

American Physical Therapy Association. Style Manual. American Physical Therapy Association, Washington, 1976.
Auger, C. P.: The Use of Reports. Archon Books, Hamden, Conn., 1975.
Barzun, J.: The Modern Researcher, ed. 3. Harcourt, Brace, Jovanovich, N.Y., 1977.
Barzun, J.: Simple and Direct: A Rhetoric for Writers. Harper and Row, N.Y., 1975.
A Manual of Style, ed. 12. University of Chicago Press, Chicago, 1969.
Campbell, W. G., and Ballou, S. V.: Form and Style, ed. 4. Houghton Mifflin, Boston, 1974.
Cordasco, F., and Gatner, E.: Research and Report Writing. Littlefield-Adams, Totowa, 1974.
DeBakey, L.: Competent medical exposition: The need and the attainment. Bull. Am. Col. Surg. 52(2):85, 1967.
Ethridge, D. A., and McSweeney, M.: Research in occupational therapy part VI: research writing. Am. J. Occup. Ther. 25(4):210, 1971.
Fishbein, M.: Medical Writing: The Technic and the Art. Charles C Thomas, Springfield, Ill., 1972.
Hutchison, H. D.: The Hutchison Guide to Writing Research Papers. Glencoe Press, N.Y., 1973.
Snyder, V. M.: The Graduate Thesis: The Complete Guide to Planning and Preparation. Pitman, N.Y., 1973.
Turabian, K. L.: A Manual for Writers, ed. 4. The University of Chicago Press, Chicago, 1973.

Appendix A

OUTLINE FOR WRITING A RESEARCH PROTOCOL

1. Long-range goal:
2. Immediate purpose:
3. Specific question(s) to be answered by this study:
4. Research hypothesis(es):
5. Null hypothesis(es):
6. Definitions of critical terms:
7. Assumptions and postulates unique to this study:
8. Type of study:
9. Population:
10. Sample:
11. Independent variable(s):
12. Dependent variable(s):
13. Potential error variables and their controls:
14. Research design (as applicable):
15. Level of measurement:
16. Measurement tool:
17. Statistical tools:
18. Procedure (where is data, how will it be obtained, how will it be used, etc.):
19. Results:
20. Clinical value (interpretation):
21. Anticipated problems:

Appendix B

Reconstructed Protocol for article by A. Jean Ayres, "Effect of Sensory Integrative Therapy on the Coordination of Children with Choreoathetoid Movements."*

1. *Long-term goal:* To develop a comprehensive program of sensory integrative therapy which will include detailed methods of both evaluation and treatment. The scope and limitations of the application of sensory integrative therapy will be defined (1,2,4,5).
2. *Immediate purpose:* To determine if sensory integrative therapy favorably affects disorders which are primarily neuromuscular in origin (1). The fact that sensory and motor are two aspects of one system gives some support to this purpose (2).
3. *Specific question to be answered by this study:* What is the effect of sensory integrative therapy on the coordination of children with choreoathetoid movements? (title of article)
4. *Research hypothesis:* The eye-hand coordination of children with minimal brain dysfunction resulting in learning disorders, sensory integrative dysfunction, and choreoathetosis will improve with sensory integrative therapy (3).
5. *Null hypothesis:* There will be no significant difference between scores on the motor accuracy test of choreoathetotic children given sensory integrative therapy one-half hour daily for six months and scores of choreoathetotic children who did not receive such therapy (3,5,7).

---

*Numbers in parentheses refer to paragraphs in the article.

6. *Definitions*

sensory integrative therapy: the article refers to the literature for this definition (6).

choreoathetosis: score on the Schilder's arm test (4).

7. *Assumptions:*
   a. The 54 children were randomly assigned to experimental and control groups (5).
   b. The Schilder's arm test correctly identifies choreoathetosis (4).
   c. Thirty minutes of therapy daily for six months is a therapeutic dose of the treatment (5).
   d. There will be no bias on the part of the classroom teachers for or against the control group (5).
   e. There will be no effective contamination of the control group by the experimental group (5).

   The textbook author is not familiar enough with sensory integrative therapy to specify postulates.

8. *Type of study:* experimental (5,11).

9. *Population:* Children around age 99 months $\pm$ 10, of normal intelligence, who are learning disabled and have mild choreoathetosis (4, Table 1).

10. *Sample:* 54 children about 99 $\pm$ months of age, most of normal intelligence who are learning disabled and who have mild choreoathetosis (4, Table 1).

11. *Independent variable:* sensory integrative therapy, individually or in pairs, one half-hour daily for about six months (5).

12. *Dependent variable:* motor accuracy test of the So. Calif. Sensory Integration Tests. Repeated measures (pre and post treatment) approximately one year apart (7).

13. *Potential error variables and their control:* age, sex, IQ—randomization assumed (Table 1); level of choreoathetosis—only mild cases admitted to study (4); cultural and family background—only control is that they are in public school special education programs (4).

14. *Research design:* two treatment groups, two independent samples (5) (randomization assumed)

15. *Level of measurement:* Metric (length) (7)

16. *Measurement tool:* linear planimeter

17. *Statistical tools*

Descriptive: mean and standard direction (7–10,12)

Correlational: none

Predictive: *t* test, one-tailed (11), Table 2.)

18. *Procedure:*
   a. Identify sample with Schilder's test (4)

b. Divide sample into experimental and control groups (5)
c. Administer motor accuracy test (7)
d. Experimental group given sensory integrative therapy in prescribed place, frequency, intensity (5,6); control group continues special education (5)
e. Repeat dependent variable, criterion measure (7)
f. Reduce data with descriptive statistics (8–10,12)
g. Perform predictive statistical test (11)
h. Interpret results (13–15)
i. Write report; submit to *American Journal of Occupational Therapy* for publication.

19. *Results:* For the more accurate hand, the null hypothesis is rejected and the alternate is supported weakly, $p < .058$ (11). For the less accurate hand the null hypothesis cannot be rejected although the results approached significance, $p < .061$ (11).

20. *Clinical value:* The long-range and immediate goals and the research hypothesis of this study are weakly supported by the data and continued study in this area is encouraged by these results (8–15). The fact that patients in the sample had disabilities other than choreoathetosis confused the interpretation (13). Where this factor has been controlled the results were more encouraging (14).

21. *Anticipated problems:* not identified in the paper but were undoubtedly in Dr. Ayres thinking as she prepared her original protocol.

Appendix C

REPRINTS OF RESEARCH ARTICLES

1. Aldag, J. C., and Martin, M. F.: Physical Therapist Assistant Selection and Academic Success
2. Ayres, A. J.: Effect of Sensory Integrative Therapy on the Coordination of Children with Choreoathetoid Movements
3. Bell, E., Jurek, K., and Wilson, T.: Hand Skill Measurement: A Gauge for Treatment
4. Carter, R. E., and Campbell, S. K.: Early Neuromuscular Development of the Premature Infant
5. Houser, C. R., and Johnson, D. M.: Breathing Exercise for Children with Pseudohypertrophic Muscular Dystrophy
6. Kielhofner, G.: Temporal Adaptation: A Conceptual Framework for Occupational Therapy
7. Montgomery, P., and Richter, E.: Effect of Sensory Integrative Therapy on the Neuromotor Development of Retarded Children
8. Payton, O. D., and Kemp, K. V.: Distribution of Peripheral Neuropathy in Diabetic Amputees
9. Tanigawa, M. C.: Comparison of the Hold-Relax Procedures and Passive Mobilization on Increasing Muscle Length
10. Tyler, N. B., and Kogan, K. L.: Reduction of Stress between Mothers and their Handicapped Children

PHYSICAL THERAPIST ASSISTANT SELECTION
AND ACADEMIC SUCCESS*

Jean C. Aldag, Ph.D., and Marjorie F. Martin, M.S.

Assessment of a standardized test as one criterion for student admission to a physical therapist assistant program is made. Comparisons are made of ACT scores between the physical therapist assistant and associate degree nurse, and the physical therapist assistant and the practical nurse. A correlation matrix was used to analyze data with differences among the three groups determined by t test computation. This sample supports a positive correlation of ACT test scores with graduation grade point average. The means show no significant difference between the two associate degree programs and a significant difference between the associate degree programs and the practical nurse program.

1. As community college programs develop for physical therapist assistants, a substantial number of prospective applicants must be considered for a limited number of class positions. Admission groups are forced to establish criteria to predict the applicant's potential success that are realistic and consistent with the equal education opportunities expressed in community college philosophies. One method to

---

*Reprinted from *Physical Therapy* (55:747–750,1975) with permission of the American Physical Therapy Association.

help assure success is to use standardized tests to assist in student selection. The use of a particular standardized test as an admission criterion for the physical therapist assistant student is examined after a four-year period of use.

2.   The American College Testing program (ACT) is one of the two most widely used admissions testing programs in community colleges and is reported to have value for student selection.[1-3] The ACT results consist of four subtest scores, one each for English, mathematics, social science, and natural science, in addition to a composite score representative of the four subtests.

3.   At Illinois Central College, admission criteria for the physical therapist assistant program were developed based on experience with admissions to other two-year health occupation associate degree programs. The ACT test was used, as well as high school rank, to determine eligibility for admission and was the same for all associate degree programs in 1968. The community college also established admission criteria to its one-year certificate programs which were less rigorous than those for associate degree programs. All applicants who did not meet the criteria initially were given an opportunity to qualify for admission by completing an outlined program of academic study in the community college with a grade point average of C or better. All student admissions were processed in a uniform manner to maintain as much objectivity as possible.

4.   The purpose of the study was to assess the following hypotheses:
1. The ACT scores for the physical therapist assistant group are positively correlated with graduation grade point average.
2. The ACT composite scores for the physical therapist assistant graduation group are significantly higher than the ACT composite scores for the dropout group.
3. Physical therapist assistant and associate degree nursing ACT scores are not significantly different.
4. Physical therapist assistant and associate degree nursing ACT scores are significantly higher than practical nurse certificate student ACT scores.

METHOD

Sample

5.   The physical therapist assistant, associate degree nurse, and practical nurse certificate samples were admitted to the community college programs from 1968 to 1972. During this interval, 104 students were admitted to the physical therapist assistant program, 251 to the

157

associate degree nurse program, and 311 to the practical nurse program. Of the 104 physical therapist assistant students admitted, 69 or 66 percent received the Associate of Applied Science Degree by June of 1974. Of the 251 associate degree nursing students admitted, 188 (75%) received the Associate of Applied Science Degree by June 1974. Of the 311 practical nursing students admitted, 262 (84%) received the certificate by June 1974.

Data Collection and Analysis

6. From the students' permanent record, the ACT subtest and composite scores, physical therapist assistant (PTA) course grades, graduation status, and final grade point average were obtained and coded for computer analysis. The correlation matrix for the physical therapist assistant variables reported in Table 1 was developed using a missing data product moment correlation program. The missing data program was necessary because each individual did not complete all variables. As the matrix involved a large number of correlations and . the predictions were 1 tail, the significant level of probability was established at .01, or $r = >.29$. The independent variable means, range, and standard deviations were computed for the physical therapist assistant (PTA), associate degree nurse (ADN), and practical nurse (PN) and are reported in Table 2. To determine the differences in the three group means, t tests were computed for the ACT scores and are reported in Table 3. The .01 level of probability was established with a t test of 2.575 or greater accepted as significant.

RESULTS AND DISCUSSION

7. The ACT subtest and composite scores reported in Table 1 all correlated significantly with the college graduation grade point average. The correlations ranged from $r = .36$ to $r = .49$ and were consistent with those reported in the literature.[2] The findings support the feasibility of using ACT test scores as one of the variables in predicting the academic success of the applicants upon graduation.
8. The ACT subtests were not significantly correlated with the physical therapist assistant course grades with the exception of the natural science and the final semester course PTA 201 grades where $r = .29$. The composite test score correlated significantly with both sophomore courses PTA 200 and 201. Using the ACT to predict individual course grades seems to be limited particularly in the freshman year.
9. The correlation of the ACT and grade point average was significant

158

Table 1. Correlation matrix for physical therapist assistant variables for a community college sample

Variable No.	1	2	3	4	5	6	7	8	9	10	11
1 — ACT English	—										
2 — ACT Mathematics	.53										
3 — ACT Social Sciences	.52	.48									
4 — ACT Natural Science	.61	.59	.59								
5 — ACT Composite Score	.78	.80	.81	.86							
6 — Grade Point Average	-.36	.40	.37	.46	.49						
7 — Age	.28	.26	.08	.12	.21	-.10					
8 — PTA 110—Foundations P.T. Assistance	.20	.20	.16	.19	.23	.73	-.19				
9 — PTA 120—Foundations P.T. Assistance	.18	.24	.22	.18	.27	.72	.02	.58			
10 — PTA 200—Foundations P.T. Assistance	.24	.26	.20	.28	.31	.71	-.09	.52	.56		
11 — PTA 201—Foundation P.T. Assistance	.13	.28	.26	.29	.31	.71	-.10	.51	.55	.66	

Sig. 01 ≥ .29

Table 2. Range, mean, and standard deviation of independent variables for associate degree nurse, practical nurse, and physical therapy assistant groups

Variable	ADN			PN			PTA		
	Range	Mean	S.D.	Range	Mean	S.D.	Range	Mean	S.D.
English	08–30	20.15	7.70	01–24	15.54	4.43	09–26	19.10	3.75
Mathematics	04–30	17.60	5.59	01–26	12.98	3.67	01–28	17.84	5.65
Social Science	06–29	20.39	5.70	05–27	14.37	5.89	04–28	18.59	5.40
Natural Science	10–30	20.32	5.20	03–28	15.59	4.78	03–30	19.52	5.24
Composite	07–33	19.74	3.98	07–28	14.73	3.74	07–27	18.92	4.19
Age	17–57	24.15	7.22	17–55	26.48	9.88	17–43	19.40	4.35

Table 3. t values for the means of the variables between physical therapist assistant, associate degree nursing, and practical nursing student groups

Independent Variable	PTA ADN	PTA PN	ADN PN
ACT English	1.121	4.497[a]	5.324[a]
ACT Mathematics	.246	5.502[a]	6.362[a]
ACT Social Science	2.340	5.113[a]	7.431[a]
ACT Natural Science	.854	4.379[a]	6.011[a]
ACT Composite	1.000	5.249[a]	7.304[a]

[a] $t \geq$ Sig. .01

for that portion of the students admitted who completed the program by graduation. To determine if the ACT was useful in predicting graduation or dropout, a t test was computed for the composite scores for the dropout and graduation groups. The mean for the dropout group was 18.121, with a standard deviation of 4.1435. For the graduation group, the mean was 19.3181 and the standard deviation, 4.1675. The t test of 2.7216 was significant at the .01 level with the graduation group mean higher than the dropout group mean.

10. Although the mean for the composite score for the graduation group was significantly higher than the composite mean for the dropout group, the magnitude of the difference was a modest 1.20 points. In addition, 20 percent of the dropout group had ACT composite scores of 22 or higher, and 20 percent of the graduation group had ACT composite scores of 15 or lower. For practical purposes, the ACT should be used cautiously in predicting academic success. The correlations of .36 to .49 account for a modest portion of variance, and undoubtedly the

interplay of ability, motivation, interest, and life circumstances has an impact on whether the student drops out or graduates from an academic program.

11. The range, mean, and standard deviation for each group are given in Table 2 for the independent variables. Inspection of Table 2 reveals a substantial range overlap within each group. The practice of permitting students who do not qualify for initial admission to the occupational program sequence to become admission-eligible by completing a prescribed program of study possibly contributes to the wide range of scores reported. This practice is consistent with the community college philosophy. The age of the physical therapist assistant student tends to be lower than that of either nursing group. As age is not considered a criterion for admission to any community college program, no subsequent test of significance was applied to the age variable. Inspection of Table 2 shows that the mean scores for each ACT variable tended to be lower for the practical nurse group than either of the two associate degree groups. To test if the differences were significant, t tests were computed and reported in Table 3. No significant differences were evident between the means of any of the variables for the associate degree groups of physical therapist assistants or nursing students. Both of the associate degree groups differed significantly from the certificate group of practical nurses on all of the ACT test scores. For these samples, the two associate degree groups appear to be drawn from the same population as measured by the ACT. Apparently, the practical nursing groups do differ significantly from the associate degree groups and the group admitted had lower scores as measured by the ACT. The practical nurse program is intended to be less rigorous in the academic requirements; however, 84 percent of the students graduated compared to 66 percent for the physical therapist assistant group and 75 percent for the associate degree nurse group.

SUMMARY

12. The study supports the hypothesis that ACT test scores are positively correlated with college grade point average for a sample of physical therapist assistant students. In addition, the study supports the hypothesis that ACT scores for the physical therapist assistant students and associate degree nursing students are not significantly different and that ACT scores for both groups are significantly higher than practical nurse test scores. Support was found for the hypothesis that ACT composite scores of the graduation group are higher than the dropout group for the physical therapist assistant sample. The suggestion was made, however, that motivation, interests, and life cir-

cumstances may have had a greater effect in attrition than ability as measured by the ACT tests.

REFERENCES

1. Assessing Students on the Way to College. Vol. 2, College Student Profiles: Norms for the ACT Assessment. Iowa City, American College Testing Program, 1972.
2. Assessing Students on the Way to College. Vol. 1, Technical Report for the ACT Assessment Program. Iowa City, American College Testing Program, 1973.
3. Wallace, W. L.: ACT. In Buros, O. K.: The Seventh Mental Measurement Yearbook. The Grypon Press, N.J., 1972, pp. 607.

EFFECT OF SENSORY INTEGRATIVE THERAPY ON THE COORDINATION OF CHILDREN WITH CHOREOATHETOID MOVEMENTS*

A. Jean Ayres

Learning-disabled children with deficits in sensory integration as well as choreoathetosis and who received sensory integrative therapy gained more on an eye-hand coordination test than did control children. Using a one-tailed test, levels of significance of difference between the mean gain scores of the experimental and control groups were .058 for the more accurate hand and .061 for the less accurate hand. It is not possible to determine whether the therapeutic effect was on the motor or on the sensory integrative aspect of coordination or on both.

1. Many children with minimal brain dysfunction show very mild involuntary motions when musculature is under voluntary contraction. These mild choreoathetoid movements, while not particularly noticeable under ordinary conditions, reflect a source of interference with fine motor coordination. The condition is probably a neuromuscular disorder and not a manifestation of sensory integrative dysfunction (paper in preparation). If this is the case, then the question

*Reprinted with permission of the American Occupational Therapy Association, Inc., from the *American Journal of Occupational Therapy* 31(5):291-293, 1977.

arises: Is the choreoathetoid state apt to improve with sensory integrative therapy?

2.   While sensory integrative therapy is designed to enhance sensory integration rather than neuromuscular coordination, many of the sensory integrative procedures are similar to those employed in treatment of neuromuscular conditions. The emphasis on co-contraction of antagonistic muscles and other sustained strong contraction of postural muscles in order to provide a given type of proprioceptive input might reasonably also influence mechanisms of motor output. Furthermore, since the sensorimotor system tends to function as a whole, it is reasonable to expect better functioning in one domain to enhance functioning in a related domain.

3.   The following hypothesis was posed and tested: The eye-hand coordination of children with minimal brain dysfunction resulting in learning disorders, sensory integrative dysfunction, and choreoathetosis will improve with sensory integrative therapy.

METHOD

4.   This investigation was part of a larger study testing the effect of sensory integrative therapy on the academic achievement of learning-disabled children. The subjects of the more extensive project were 94 public school children with learning disorders. All were receiving special education. From this larger sample, the 54 children with mild choreoathetosis were selected to test the hypothesis stated above. The choreoathetoid movements were judged during the execution of Schilder's arm extension test.[1] As applied in this situation, with the examiner the child counted aloud to 20 while standing with feet together, arms outstretched, fingers abducted, and eyes closed. The examiner observed any involuntary motion of a choreoathetoid quality present in the fingers of the child.

5.   Thirty-one of the 54 children composed an experimental group that was taken from special education classes, individually or in pairs, for one-half hour each day to receive sensory integrative therapy for about six months over a one-year period; 23 constituted a control group and received the equivalent, in time, of special education by remaining in their classrooms. The age, sex distribution, and IQs of the two groups are shown in Table 1.

6.   The primary objective of the therapeutic program of the larger study was enhancement of the sensory integrative basis of academic learning; improvement of coordination was not a major concern in itself. Because of the prevalence of vestibular system disorder in the children, therapy for the experimental group was focused on ameliora-

164

Table 1. Age, intelligence quotient (IQ), and sex distribution of children in experimental and control groups

	Experimental	Control
Age in Months:		
Mean	98.81	100.91
Standard Deviation	12.28	9.97
IQ:		
Mean	99.87	100.30
Standard Deviation	15.21	18.08
Sex:		
Number of Females	5	7
Number of Males	26	16
Total Number	31	23

tion of that deficit. Some emphasis was placed on gross motor planning for those with developmental apraxia, but there was practically no activity involving fine motor or eye-hand coordination included in the therapeutic program. A more complete description of the treatment rationale and its effect on academic achievement may be found elsewhere.[2,3]

7.   Experimental and control subjects were administered the Motor Accuracy Test of the Southern California Sensory Integration Tests[4] both before the therapeutic program and again approximately one year later. That test requires the subject to draw a pencil line over a long, curved standard guide line. The degree of accuracy of the subject's performance is measured and scored. Because the range of standard deviation (SD) scores on the Motor Accuracy Test tends to be inordinately wide, the scores were converted to a more normal distribution by using a logarithmic scale. When this scale was used there was no change of SD scores as determined by use of the test manual for those scores falling between plus or minus 1.5 standard deviations, but scores falling beyond those points tended to show less deviation from the mean. A score of -3.0 SD became -2.5 SD; a score of -4.0 SD became -3.0 SD; and a score of -7.0 SD became -4.0 SD. The difference between pre- and post-test scores was computed for both right and left hands.

RESULTS

8.   The means, standard deviations, and ranges of initial SD scores and amount of change in SD scores after one year for both experimental and control groups are shown in Table 2. As can be seen from the table,

Table 2. Initial motor accuracy (MAC) standard deviation (SD) scores of experimental and control groups, amount of change in scores, and significance of difference between the groups' mean (Mn) change scores

	Initial MAC Mn/SD	SD Scores Range	Change in MAC Scores Mn/SD	t Value	Degrees of Freedom	One-tailed Probability
More Accurate Hand:						
Experimental Group	−2.14/1.10	−4.2 to −0.1	−0.14/1.13	1.60	47.85	.058
Control Group	−1.18/1.02	−3.5 to −0.4	−0.62/1.02			
Less Accurate Hand:						
Experimental Group	−1.73/1.07	−3.7 to +0.3	−0.50/1.08	1.57	49.22	.061
Control Group	−1.28/1.22	−4.3 to +0.2	−0.94/0.92			

before conducting the study, the experimental group's average coordination of both more and less accurate hands was somewhat lower than that of the control group. The fact that the standard deviation of the SD scores was greater than 1.0 indicates the variance in both of these groups was greater than that of the normative population.

9. Since the eye-hand skill of these poorly coordinated children varied from the normative growth rate, the expected change due to maturation alone would be something less than 0.0 SD. This was the case. Both groups had lower mean motor accuracy (MAC) SD scores on post-testing than in pre-testing. The lower SD score does not necessarily indicate a lower raw score, for considerable increase in raw score is expected during a year's normal growth just to maintain the same SD.

10. While the mean gain of the control group's more accurate hand was so little it resulted in a loss of nearly two-thirds of a SD, the comparable gain of the group receiving therapy was the equivalent of a little less than 1 SD. The less accurate hands of both groups gained less (a greater SD loss) than the more accurate hands, although the experimental group gained more than did the control group.

11. Since it was hypothesized that treatment would improve eye-hand coordination, a one-tailed t-test was used to determine the significance of difference between the mean gain scores. For the more accurate hand, the difference was significant at the .058 level; and for the less accurate hand, the difference was significant at the .061 level.

12. There is a reasonable probability that sensory integrative therapy did improve the eye-hand coordination of some, but not all, members of the experimental group, although the difference in group means did not reach the classically acceptable level of significance. The fact that the SD of the change scores was as much as the SD of the pre-test scores indicates considerable variability among the subjects; some improved appreciably, while others had lower post-test raw scores than pre-test raw scores. Some of the variability may be ascribed to the difficulty that learning-disabled children experience in attending carefully to a demanding task, thereby reducing the reliability of their test scores. The large variations in change increase the difficulty in demonstrating statistically significant changes.

DISCUSSION

13. Since all of the children in this sample had sensory integration deficits in addition to the dyskinesia, it is not possible to differentiate the effect of therapy on the choreoathetoid state from that on integration of sensory input. Choreoathetosis is seen as a problem of insuffi-

167

cient motor inhibition. Eye-hand coordination is dependent not only upon neuromuscular conditions but also upon integration of visual, vestibular, and somatosensory input. In the larger population of 96 (46 experimental and 50 control) subjects, which included children with sensory integrative deficits as well as the children of this study who had choreoathetosis, t-values representing the mean gain of the experimental group that received therapy over the gain of the control group were statistically significant ($p = <.05$, one-tailed test) for the less accurate hand. Difference in mean gains for the more accurate hand did not reach the level of statistical significance. The data of this study do not, in themselves, clarify the question of whether therapy reduced the disordered motor problem or enhanced the sensory integrative basis of eye-hand coordination.

14. Studies on the effect of vestibular stimulation on motor function of children without the sensory integrative problems classically found in the learning-disabled child suggest therapy designed to enhance vestibular system function has a considerable positive effect on motor performance, especially in postural-ocular responses.[5-8] However, Casler[9] failed to find such an effect on normal, full-term institutionalized infants.

15. While sensory integrative therapy may or may not reduce the motor release condition, there may be enough other mechanisms involved in coordination that are enhanced through therapy to enable improvement of the final eye-hand motor skill in the child with mild choreoathetosis.

ACKNOWLEDGMENTS

This research was supported by grants from the Center for the Study of Sensory Integrative Dysfunction and the Valentine-Kline Foundation. The following public school districts cooperated in the study: Manhattan Beach City, Redondo Beach City, and Torrance Unified. Florence Davis and Edward T. Dawson assisted the author in testing and treating. Mary A. Silberzahn assisted in post-testing. Dr. Thomas J. Reynolds and Robert Cudeck served as statisticians. Reprint requests should be directed to the Center for the Study of Sensory Integrative Dysfunction, 201 South Lake Avenue, Room 311, Pasadena, California 91101.

REFERENCES

1. Schilder, P.: Contributions to Developmental Neuropsychiatry. International Universities Press, New York, 1964.

2. Ayres, A. J.: Sensory Integration and Learning Disorders. Western Psychological Services, Los Angeles, 1972.
3. Ayres, A. J.: Improving academic scores through sensory integration. J. Learn. Disabil. 5:338, 1972.
4. Ayres, A. J.: Southern California Sensory Integration Tests. Western Psychological Services, Los Angeles, 1972.
5. Chee, F. K. W., et al.: Effects of vestibular stimulation on motor performance in normal and cerebral palsied children. Paper presented at the 89th Annual Session of the American Association of Anatomists, Louisville, Kentucky, April 1976.
6. Gregg, C. L., et al.: The relative efficacy of vestibular-proprioceptive stimulation and the upright position in enhancing visual pursuits in neonates. Child. Dev. 47:309, 1976.
7. Kantner, R. M., et al.: Effects of vestibular stimulation on nystagmus response and motor performance in the developmentally delayed infant. Phys. Ther. 56:414, 1976.
8. Cornell, E. H. and Gottfried, A. W.: Intervention with premature infants. Child. Dev. 47:32, 1976.
9. Casler, L.: Supplementary auditory and vestibular stimulation: Effects on institutionalized infants. J. Exp. Child Psychol. 19:456, 1975.

HAND SKILL MEASUREMENT:
A GAUGE FOR TREATMENT*

Esther Bell, Kathleen Jurek, and Thelma Wilson

Objective measurements of performance are vital with the increasing necessity to justify the need for occupational therapy services, and to conduct studies that measure the effectiveness of treatment procedures. This paper reports on a measurement of hand skill that was standardized by comparing hand skill performance among the able-bodied, or normal, population. The performance on this test of patients with various types of disabilities and the implications for treatment are discussed. For the paraplegic, the hand skill test indicates the need for occupational therapy services; for the quadriplegic, the test measures the effectiveness of functional orthotic devices; and for the hemiplegic, the hand skill test determines the potential for success in one aspect of self-care, dressing.

1. The occupational therapist is frequently requested to make an objective judgment of a patient's hand skill based upon subjective clinical observations. Although occupational therapy provides an ideal setting in which to observe hand skill performance, subjective observations results in statements that are prefaced by "probably" or "it appears,"

---

*Reprinted with permission of the American Occupational Therapy Association, Inc., from the *American Journal of Occupational Therapy* 30(2):80–86, 1976. Photographs have been omitted.

since subjective observations are not legally defensible unless prefaced by these statements. Such indecisive statements do not sound significant when reported to the doctor, other allied health personnel, or third-party carriers, although the observations may be correct. Subjective observations cannot be used in research studies to measure the effectiveness of treatment techniques. For these reasons, the occupational therapy department at the Texas Rehabilitation Hospital developed an objective standardized test of hand skill, called the Physical Capacities Evaluation of Hand Skill (PCE).

BACKGROUND

2.   In use at this hospital for ten years, the PCE has proved invaluable in presenting the major clinical observations of hand performance in a measurable form. The test was developed originally as a pre-vocational tool,[1] but now it is effective in measuring the status of hand skill regardless of vocational potential, and in determining the need for occupational therapy services. The test measures progress toward fulfilling treatment goals, thereby determining the effectiveness of the treatment, and the need for further, or for cessation of, treatment. Data have been gathered to determine the norms for three disability groups—paraplegia, left hemiplegia, and right hemiplegia—so that the norms of individuals with one of these disabilities can be compared both to the norms for able-bodied individuals and to others with the same disability. A correlation was established between results of the test and the success of the rehabilitation process for the left and right hemiplegic. These test results can thus be used to predict success in rehabilitation.

3.   Since the PCE is based upon able-bodied norms, its value is not limited to those with a physical disability. Not all individuals who possess normal musculature have normal skills, nor do they have equal skill in each hand. This test can detect minor deviations in hand skill that indicate a need for the services of the occupational therapist.

DESCRIPTION OF THE PCE TEST*

4.   The PCE test battery is composed of five unilateral hand skill tests, seven bilateral hand skill tests, and a dynamometer reading. The unilateral tests measure gross cylindrical or extrinsic grasp and release, intrinsic grasp and release, tripod or jawchuck prehension, finger tip pinch and manipulation, and fingernail pinch. The bilateral

---

*Tests appear at the end of this article.

171

tests measure similar types of hand skill. The tests were designed for ease of accomplishment even by individuals who had some physical involvement of the hands. The tests are timed for either a specified period or for completion of the task because one of the components of skill is speed.[2]

5.   The scores for each of the subtests were standardized by using a sample population of 50 subjects. The 30 women and 20 men included hospital employees and volunteers, or were from patients' families and community church groups. Their age range was from 19 to 68 years. This sample represented a variety of occupations and three ethnic groups: black, white, and Latin American.

6.   The mean for each test was set at a standard score of 100 with two standard deviations above the mean set at 130, and two standard deviations below the mean set at 70. This range is considered the normal or "able-bodied" range. Standard deviations were used to project the scores to zero with a score of 10 being six standard deviations below the mean.

7.   The tests measure only hand skill—not the ability to follow directions, use of the correct pattern of hand motion, arm reach, or endurance. Directions are verbal but the tests are also demonstrated. Practice time is allowed. The examinee is shown the correct hand pattern commonly used in performing the task but is instructed to experiment as necessary to find his/her best method before timing is started. If an inefficient pattern of hand motion is used, the examinee will usually perform more slowly and thus be penalized by a low score. The test table is placed at an advantageous working height and the test boards are positioned to accommodate the examinee's best arm reach. The test is administered in small time segments if endurance proves to be a problem. Notations are kept on deviate methods of performing the test but are not part of the scoring since the test measures hand skill under optimum performance conditions.

8.   When test results above and below 70 are graphed with contrasting colored pencils, deficits can be spotted quickly. The five subtests for each hand and the seven bilateral tests are averaged to determine an average skill score for the right, for the left, and for both hands.

PERFORMANCE OF PATIENTS IN THREE DISABILITY CATEGORIES

Paraplegia

9.   Since individuals who are paraplegic as a result of spinal cord injury do not have upper extremity neurological involvement, it could be

assumed that their hand skill would be comparable to that of the sample or normal population. This assumption proved to be false. Eighty paraplegic subjects with normal upper extremity musculature were tested for average hand skill performance. The sample ranged in age from 19 to 57 years with twice as many men as women. The range of vocational and cultural backgrounds was similar to that represented in the able-bodied population used to develop the norms for the PCE. The length of time from onset of disability in the paraplegic sample population varied from two months to six years. Those close to onset had been involved in an active rehabilitation program for at least one month before being tested. The average score on the five skill tests with the right and with the left hand for this group was 85, or 15 points below the mean of 100 (Fig. 1). Bilateral test scores were not compared.

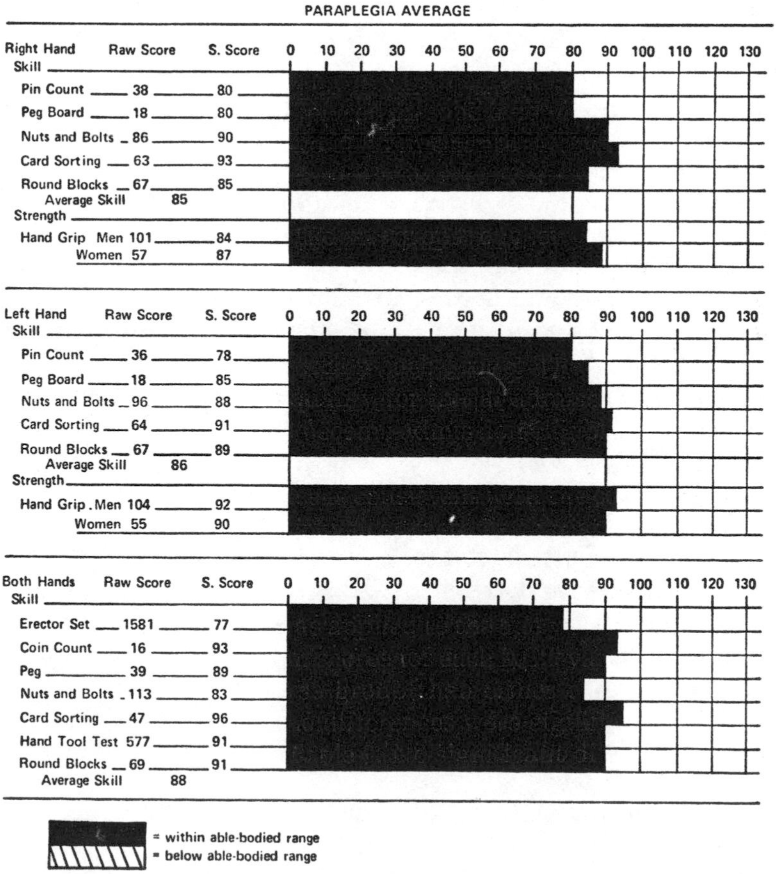

Figure 1. Average hand skill for paraplegic subjects

10. The reasons for the 15-point difference could be related to the effects of bed rest, sensory deprivation, or psychological problems.[3] The psychological problems encountered in adjusting to a disability could explain the subjects' lack of competitiveness in the test situation. For example, they seemed unaware that they were being timed even when reminded, neither were they interested in their test results nor in improving their scores.

11. Since the paraplegic is frequently expected to return to a job where he uses his hands, the PCE is used as a screening device to determine the need for further treatment. If the subject scores average or above on hand skill, further treatment is not recommended. If the subject scores lower than average, occupational therapy is recommended with emphasis on increasing hand skill, speed, initiative, and competitiveness in work. When retested one month later after receiving occupational therapy, reasonable gains in hand skill can be seen. Correlation of these gains with later success in employment has not been completed.

Quadriplegia

12. When an individual with quadriplegia from a cervical cord lesion has some use of the hands, either through tenodesis action or through use of residual finger musculature, the occupational therapist often evaluates the individual's success in using this hand pattern for functional purposes. The occupational therapist also frequently evaluates the potential for improving the individual's function through use of a functional orthosis, such as a simple opponens or wrist-driven finger-flexion orthosis. The PCE can be used to test hand skill both with and without an orthosis and can provide a graphic comparison of hand function. Test results indicate that sometimes the orthosis increases skill, sometimes it decreases skill, and in some instances the skill in one pattern of hand use is increased by an orthosis but skill in another pattern of hand use is decreased. The comparison of test results obtained with and without an orthosis can be used to guide both the therapist and the quadriplegic individual in choosing the most effective functional orthosis or in the decision to use no orthosis.

Hemiplegia

13. From necessity individuals with hemiplegia frequently perform all activities of daily living with only one hand. It is therefore important to develop maximum skill in the one functioning hand. The PCE pro-

174

vides a useful tool with which to measure the degree of skill in the functioning upper extremity.

14.   Forty-four hemiplegic subjects who suffered a cerebral vascular accident with residual paralysis of the right arm were studied to determine the average skill performance of the left extremity on the PCE. The subjects studied ranged in age from 30 to 75 years with a mean age of 50 years. There were equal numbers of men and women. All were previously right-handed. The nondominant left hand was tested. The average score on the five skill tests for the left hand for this group was 68 compared to the normal mean of 100 (Fig. 2), which placed them in the low able-bodied range. This low performance was attributed to age, poor health, or to disuse.

15.   Fifty patients who suffered a cerebral vascular accident with residual paralysis of their nondominant left arm were studied to determine the degree of their hand skills. These subjects were between 20 and 82 years of age with a mean age of 51 years. There were equal numbers of men and women. The right hand was tested on the five skill tests. The subjects' average score was 44 (Fig. 3), far below the normal mean of 100 and the normal able-bodied range of 70 to 130.

16.   Causes for this low performance on hand skill may be similar to those for the right hemiplegic, that is, age, disuse, and poor health, but this does not explain why the right hemiplegic scores 68, while the left hemiplegic scores only 44. Some of the other problems identified with left hemiplegia such as a poor time sense, poor motor planning, or perceptual difficulties may be important factors contributing to the test results. [4-6] The poor sense of time may be reflected in the typical pattern seen in the test results of a left hemiplegic whose scores on the

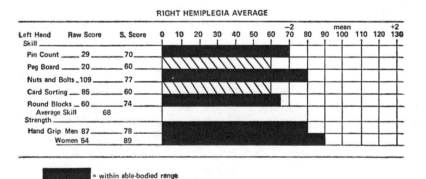

Figure 2. Average hand skill for right hemiplegic subjects

175

Right Hand	Raw Score	S. Score	0	10	20	30	40	50	60	−2 70	80	90	mean 100	110	120	+2 130
Skill																
Pin Count	25	60														
Peg Board	18	50														
Nuts and Bolts	145	11														
Card Sorting	115	16														
Round Blocks	47	57														
Average Skill		44														
Strength																
Hand Grip Men	74	67														
Women	46	75														

= within able-bodied range
= below able-bodied range

Figure 3. Average hand skill for left hemiplegic subjects

nuts and bolts and card sorting were the lowest of those tested. Also, these two tests are the only tests that are timed to completion. Results are higher on the other three tests timed for one minute each. Poor awareness of time may not penalize the subject as much in the short one-minute time period as it does in a longer time period where tests are timed to completion.

17.   Working to develop skill of the noninvolved right hand of a left hemiplegic individual is not always stressed as a treatment aim for occupational therapy and yet results on the PCE indicate that it is a very important need, probably even more so than in the right hemiplegic. The left hemiplegic individual is attempting to learn one-handed skills with a hand that scores very low in skill. Studies indicate that left hemiplegic subjects do not often succeed in rehabilitation.[6] Low hand skill could be one of the contributing factors.

THE PCE USED AS A PREDICTOR OF SUCCESS

18.   A review of the literature indicates that various studies were conducted in an attempt to find a psychological or perceptual test that would indicate the degree of potential for successful rehabilitation of the hemiplegic individual,[6-8] but as yet no definite correlations have been found. A study using the performance portion of the Wechsler Adult Intelligence Scale suggests that this did provide some predictive ability but only when the initial self-care status was very low.[9] During a period of five years, the occupational therapy staff used two tests in an attempt to determine whether or not a relationship existed between success in learning activities of daily living and one of the following factors; age, scores on a perception test, or scores on the Bender-Gestalt Test. No strong correlations were found.

176

19. A follow-up study of 30 subjects with hemiplegia was conducted to determine whether or not the PCE battery of tests could serve as a useful predictor of success in learning the activities of daily living.

20. Dressing was identified as the element of self-care to be measured since one-handed dressing requires more retraining than most other aspects of self-care. Dressing was rated on a scale of 1 to 5: 1. Unable to dress self; 2. dressed partially but was forgetful or resistive; 3. able to dress except for difficulty with a few small items; 4. able to dress but had minor difficulty or was slow; 5. able to dress independently with ease.

21. Since the average scores on the PCE for the sample population of 30 subjects ranged from 16 to 90, the range was divided into five segments for ease of handling. 1. 16–32; 2. 33–49; 3. 50–66; 4. 67–83; 5. 84–100.

22. When the PCE segment ratings were correlated with the dressing scale ratings, it was found that those who scored from segment 3 to 5 (50 or above on the PCE) were usually successful in learning to dress at a segment 3 or above dressing rating. The probability of those who score 50 or above on the PCE in succeeding to learn to dress, at least at a segment 3 dressing level, was tested on the conditional probability theory and a .98 probability was found. Therefore, a PCE score of 50 or above could be used as a predictor that the subject would learn to be independent in most items of dressing.

23. Since the average PCE right-hand skill score of the left hemiplegic subjects was 44, a prediction can be made that the average left hemiplegic individual probably will not learn to dress successfuly. The subject may learn the steps of dressing but will probably forget or refuse to do them at home. For the average right hemiplegic individual with a skill score of 68, a prediction can be made that the individual will learn to dress.

24. Following this study, the treatment emphasis in occupational therapy was changed. With a hemiplegic subject who scores below 50 on the PCE, a brief trial in dressing training is given. If this is unsuccessful, treatment emphasis is redirected toward developing skill of the unaffected hand. The test is readministered every three to four weeks. When the PCE score increases to 50, dressing training is begun again. Results indicate that dressing skills are then usually learned in less than one week of treatment, in contrast to the many weeks experienced in the past with generally unsuccessful results.

SUMMARY

25. The Physical Capacities Evaluation (PCE) provides an objective

method of evaluating hand skill, measuring progress, indicating the need for treatment, and can also be used for comparative studies in measuring the effectiveness of treatment procedures. With paraplegic subjects, the test can be used to indicate a need for occupational therapy to develop hand skill suitable for employment requirements. With quadriplegic subjects, the test battery may be useful to measure progress in developing skill in tenodesis function or to determine the potential value of functional orthosis. For hemiplegic subjects, the test battery indicates the need for hand skill development of the uninvolved hand before dressing training can be successful. This evaluation may also be used to identify minor problems of finger dexterity that may interfere with good performance.

26.   Tables converting raw scores on the test to standard scores are available from the authors upon request.

PIN COUNT TEST

Materials: Box of straight pins, not round headed
Directions: Examiner spreads pins out on table. Subject picks pins up one at a time and places them in pin box.
Time: One minute
Score: Number of pins picked up

HAND GRIP TEST

Materials: Use Preston Corp. #5031 dynamometer
Directions: Grip best one-handed method possible.
Score: Grip twice, take best reading.

COIN COUNT TEST

Materials: One .0889 meter (3½ inches) × .0762 meter (3 inches) snap top coin purse. Five pennies, three quarters, one dime, two nickels
Directions: Remove all coins from purse one at a time.
Time: Length of time from opening of purse to closing of purse
Score: Number of seconds

CARD SORT TEST

Materials: Stack of fifty 5 × 8 cards
Directions: *Unilateral.* Cards stacked in middle of test table. Subject

places one card on one side of center stack, then one on other side. Continue until original stack is sorted into two.

Bilateral. Right hand places card on right side of stack, left hand places card on left-hand side.

Time: Timed to completion of sort

Score: Number of seconds taken to complete

ERECTOR SET TEST

Materials: Erector Set #1½

Directions: Assemble "Bundle Truck" from picture, using screw driver provided in set. A few minutes are allowed to study the picture and pieces.

Time: To completion of task

Score: Number of seconds to complete

HAND TOOL TEST

Materials: Bennet Hand Tool Dexterity Test available from The Psychological Corporation. Use as directed.

Time: Number of seconds to complete

NUTS AND BOLTS TEST

Materials: *Unilateral.* .7620 meter (30 inches) × .1524 meter (6 inches) test board with ten .0158 meter (⅝ inch) bolts set permanently in the board so that a nut can be screwed on each bolt. Bolts are .0508 meters (2 inches) apart.

Bilateral. Bolts are in trough on one side, nuts in trough on other side. Ten holes are provided in test board to have a place to put the completed nut and bolt assembly.

Directions: *Unilateral.* Subject screws the nut on the fixed bolt until the nut is flush with the tip of the bolt. Subject places ten nuts on, then takes them off, replacing them in trough, one at a time.

Bilateral. Subject picks up bolt in one hand, nuts in other hand, and screws them together until nut is flush with tip of bolt. Place finished assembly in holes in board. Ten together, take ten apart, and replace bolt and nut to troughs.

Time: Number of seconds to complete

Score: Add time for on and off together. Repeat test and average scores.

179

PEGBOARD TEST*

Materials: .3048 meter (12 inches) × .3810 meter (15 inches) test board. Twenty-five pairs of .0047 meter (³⁄₁₆ inch) holes lined up in center of .3048 (12 inch) side. Holes are placed .0127 meter (½ inch) apart in both pairs and rows. Four troughs, .0127 meter (½ inch) deep with tapered sides, .0508 meter (2 inch) diameter holes.
Pegs: 25, .0032 meter (⅛ inch) metal pegs, .0254 (1 inch) long.
Washers: 25, hole is .0047 (³⁄₁₆ inch), outside is .0158 meter (⅝ inch).
Sleeves: 25, .0047 meter (³⁄₁₆ inch) diameter inside. Sleeve is .0158 meter (⅝ inches) tall. Place half of sleeves in right outer trough, half in left outer trough.
Directions: *Unilateral.* Subject places a peg in the closest right-hand hole with the right hand (left-hand hole with left hand), then places a washer on the peg with the same hand, followed by a sleeve on the peg with the same hand.

Bilateral. Place a peg in the right-hand hole with the right hand, washer with the left, sleeve with the right. Place a peg in the left-hand hole with the left, washer with the right, sleeve with the left.
Time: *Unilateral.* One minute timed twice

Bilateral. Two minute times twice
Score: *Unilateral.* Number of individual pieces assembled in one minute. Average two timings.

Bilateral. Number of individual pieces assembled in two minutes. Average two timings.

ROUND BLOCKS TEST

Materials: One test board, .7620 meter (30 inches) × .2032 meter (8 inches). Two rows of eight blocks each. Blocks are .0508 meter (2 inches) in diameter and .0190 meter (¾ inches) thick. Blocks are set in board in holes .0127 meter (½ inch) deep.
Directions: *Unilateral.* Right hand starts at left-hand side of board and turns blocks over one at a time, moving from left to right and from right to left on row two. Continue turning around two rows until time is called. Reverse order for left hand.

Bilateral. Right hand starts at left-hand side of board, picks up block, turns it over, left hand takes it and replaces it in hole. On second row left hand picks up block, turns it over, and right hand replaces it.
Time: One minute timed twice

---

*Similar to Purdue Pegboard but pieces are larger to allow use by those with severe hand involvement.

Score: Count number of blocks turned in one minute. Average two timings.

REFERENCES

1. Bell, E.: Development of an evaluation of physical capacities. In: Proceedings of the Annual Conference of the American Occupational Therapy Association, Denver, 1964.
2. Singer, R.: Motor Learning and Human Performance. Macmillan Co., N.Y., 1968.
3. Zubek, J.: Behavioral and physiological changes during prolonged immobilization plus perceptual deprivation. J. Abnorm. Psychol. 74:230, 1969.
4. Rosenthal, A. et al.: Correlation of perceptual factors with rehabilitation of hemiplegic patient. Arch. Phys. Med. 46:461, 1965.
5. Carroll, V.: Implications of measured visuospatial impairment in a group of left hemiplegic patients. Arch. Phys. Med. 39:55, 1958.
6. Knapp, M.: Problems in the rehabilitation of the hemiplegic patient. JAMA 169:224, 1959.
7. Knapp, M.: Results of language tests of patients with hemiplegia. Arch. Phys. Med. 43:317, 1962.
8. Lorenze, E. et al.: Psychological studies in geriatric hemiplegia. J. Am. Geriatr. Soc. 9:39, 1961.
9. Bourstrom, J., and Howard, M.: Behavioral correlates of recovery in hemiplegic patients. Arch. Phys. Med. 49:449, 1968.

EARLY NEUROMUSCULAR DEVELOPMENT
OF THE PREMATURE INFANT*

Russell E. Carter, M.P.H., and Suzann K. Campbell, Ph.D.

A case study is presented which documents the neuromuscular development of a premature infant (34–35 weeks gestation) during the first eight weeks of postnatal life. The development of postural tone, spontaneous activity, and responsiveness to stimulation is described and compared with that of the full-term infant. This information is of value to physical therapists involved in evaluation and therapeutic intervention programs for high risk infants.

1.   The motor patterns and muscle tone of the premature infant differ from those of the full-term baby in the neonatal period and early months of infancy.[1-3] In attempting to assess the presence of central nervous system deficits in premature infants examined in the Special Infant Care Clinic at North Carolina Memorial Hospital, we found that our experience and knowledge of the appropriate responses to stimulation or test procedures were frequently inadequate. While helpful, the descriptions by Saint-Anne Dargassies of the premature infant's development are primarily subjective, making difficult the determination of *degrees* of change which are appropriate during early infancy.[2,3] We, therefore, performed a longitudinal study of the neuromuscular

---

*Reprinted from *Physical Therapy* (55:1332-1340, 1975) with permission of the American Physical Therapy Association.

development of a "normal" premature infant, using objective ratings and subjective observations, to improve our ability to recognize abnormalities, as well as appropriate responses, in these infants. We described the following responses from birth to forty-two weeks postmenstrual age: muscle tone, sucking and rooting reactions and other primitive reflexes, spontaneous activity, behavioral state, and head control with the child in the prone and upright positions and when pulled to sitting from the supine position.

METHODS

Subject

2.   A white male infant, N. M., was randomly selected from the infants residing in the premature nursery at North Carolina Memorial Hospital at the time the study began. The infant's mother was twenty-four years old and had not experienced any complications during this second pregnancy. The 1,700 gram infant was the first-born of twins delivered with low forceps, occiput anterior presentation, after a four and one-half hour labor at thirty-four to thirty-five weeks gestation. Oxytocin was used as well as the epidural anesthetic, bupivicaine. Suctioning and bagging with oxygen were required to elicit respiration. The Apgar scores were 4 at one minute and 6 at five minutes. [4]

3.   The infant had mild respiratory distress during the first hours of life which resolved within the first twenty-four hours. An umbilical catheter was inserted but was removed during the first twenty-four hours. A sugar-water solution was offered during the first two days and formula was begun on day 3. On day 4, the infant appeared to be jaundiced, and a diagnosis of hyperbilirubinemia was made on day 5. Phototherapy[5] was employed in the resolution of the jaundice until day 6. On day 9, breast milk was first fed, and, on day 10, breast feeding began with formula supplementing the diet. Body temperature fluctuations were reported on day 10, with stabilization on day 12. Conditioning, the process of allowing the infant to regulate his own body temperature, was instituted at seventeen days. On day 20, the infant was removed from the incubator and placed in a crib. On day 25, he was circumcised. An electrocardiogram was performed on day 27 to rule out suspected peripheral pulmonary stenosis; normal heart sounds were reported. On day 28, N. M. was discharged home weighing 2,160 grams. His subsequent medical course was reportedly unremarkable. The infant, as well as his twin, has been followed in our Special Infant Care Clinic and at thirteen months of age, both infants appear to be normal in all respects.

183

Method of Examination

4.   The neurological examination followed a format similar to that described by Prechtl and Beintema in The Neurological Examination of the Full Term Newborn Infant[6] supplemented by the work of André-Thomas, Chesni, and Saint-Anne Dargassies.[7] Objective scores were assigned when possible. Throughout the study, consistent observation under standard conditions was attempted. These conditions were as follows:

1. *Time of Examination.* Prechtl and Beintema reported that the optimal time for an infant examination is two or three hours after a feeding[6]; this timing was also suggested for the examination of the premature infant since the infant would be less likely to be irritable or to fall asleep.[8] We adopted such a schedule for the testing of our subject.

2. *Place of Examination.* The examination was conducted in the premature nursery, under thermoneutral conditions (isolette or radiant heater). After the infant was discharged, examinations were conducted in the home in a well-lighted area of constant warm temperature.

3. *State of the Baby.* Since the physiological status of the infant is reflected in the quality of responses elicited during an examination,[9] the following behavioral states were scored and recorded during each test:

State I: Eyes closed, regular respiration, no movements
State II: Eyes closed, irregular respiration, no gross movements
State III: Eyes open, no gross movements
State IV: Eyes open, gross movements, no crying
State V: Eyes open or closed, crying
State II/IV: Eyes closed, gross movements[6,10]

During the examinations in the first five days of postnatal life, the infant was in State II/IV. Neither State III nor State IV was observed by the investigator before day 6. From that day until the end of the study, the infant was examined consistently during State III or IV.

4. *Personnel Conducting Examinations.* All examinations were conducted by the first author.

5. *Item Sequence.* The sequence of administration of the test items was the same on each day. The items in each basic test position were conducted in a sequence proceeding from least demanding to most demanding of the infant, minimizing the actual amount of handling of the infant in an effort to maintain a constant state.

6. *Testing Frequency.* The subject was examined daily through the first ten days, twice during the third week, and weekly thereafter. Because of interrupting circumstances (for example, health of the in-

fant or investigator), testing was not possible on day 4 and during the fifth week. A total of sixteen examinations was completed between birth and forty-two weeks of postmenstrual age (a chronological age of 8 weeks).

5.   Each assessment began with a three-minute observation of the spontaneous postures and motor activity of the supine infant. After this observation, reflexes and reactions were evaluated. The following rating system was used:[6, 7]

Supine

1. *Spontaneous Activity.* Observation of infant for three minutes, accounting for basic postural set, state, amount of movement, type of movement, and direction and results of movement, such as auto-elicitation of reflexes and tremors. The amount of time the child was active was scored:

    0—none
    1—spontaneous activity during less than 30 percent of the observation time
    2—infant active more than 50 percent of the observation time
    3—infant constantly active during observation with only brief pauses of inactivity (less than 10 seconds)

2. *Sucking Response.* Insertion of approximately three centimeters of the examiner's little finger into the baby's mouth. The ease or difficulty encountered in eliciting the suck was described. The strength of the suck was graded:

    0—no response
    1—one or two sucking movements in ten seconds with little lip or tongue pressure on the examiner's finger
    2—several sucking movements (3 to 6) in ten seconds with full stripping by tongue, and lip pressure on examiner's finger
    3—long sucking (6 or more) in ten seconds with full stripping by tongue, and lip pressure on examiner's finger
    4—full and uninterrupted sucking (15 seconds or more)

3. *Rooting Responses.* Elicited by lightly stroking the perioral area, the upper lip, and the lower lip with the little finger. The head was in the midline. The responses were scored:

    0—no response
    1—only lip movements toward stimulus
    2—lip and tongue movements visible, plus incomplete turning of the head
    3—full turn of the head toward stimulus
    4—full turn, with lip grasping (requiring repeated stimuli)

185

5—easily elicited full turning and lip grasping (single stimulus)

4. *Palmar Response.* Elicited by placing the examiner's index finger in the infant's palm from the ulnar side and producing a slight stretch of the flexor muscles. The response was scored:

0—no response

1—incomplete flexion of fingers, not touching examiner's finger throughout test

2—complete flexion of fingers, but only lightly touching examiner's fingers through full test (examiner may easily remove finger from infant's grasp)

3—full flexion, but maintained for less than ten seconds (examiner may raise infant's arm off mat before infant's grasp releases)

4—full flexion maintained for longer than ten seconds (infant's arm and shoulder can be raised off mat)

5—fingers strongly flexed and have to be retracted by the examiner

5. *Tonic Labyrinthine Reflex.* Posture of shoulders, arms, and legs, and possible opisthotonos when lying supine were first noted. Then the examiner placed a hand behind the infant's head and passively flexed the head to the chest. The amount of resistance to passive motion was graded:

0—floppy, no resistance to passive neck movement

1—resistance through any part of range, but easily moved through the full range

2—resistance strong in initial part of range; some resistance throughout the range which increases with increase in velocity of neck movement

3—head and neck firmly press into examiner's hand; difficult to initiate movement but full range possible; resistance throughout the range

4—head and neck firmly press into examiner's hand, trunk arching; difficult to passively move head and neck, and full range is not possible without strong effort by examiner

6. *Muscle Tone.* Resistance to passive movement of the arms and legs was scored:

0—floppy

1—resistance to passive motion, but falls back to initial position

2—resistance through full range, with immediate rapid return to position

3—resists passive motion, restricted range, immediate return to initial position

7. *Asymmetrical Tonic Neck Reflex.* First the examiner tried to elicit active head rotation to one side and then to the other by visual distraction. If active head rotation could not be obtained, the examiner passively turned the head to one side, and then to the other. After the head was rotated, a description of the infant's posture was recorded.

8. *Pull to Sit.* The examiner gradually pulled the infant from supine to sitting while supporting the infant by the upper arms and shoulders. The movement was scored:

0—head passively hangs; no attempt to right head

1—head hangs down, but infant attempts to assist slightly with shoulders and neck

2—head hangs down through the first 60 degrees, then infant can right head

3—head hangs down through the first 45 degrees, then infant can right head

4—infant cannot initiate, but brings head up through most of the range

5—infant actively pulls to sit, using head and arms

9. *Head Control and Posture When Sitting.* The examiner rated the sitting posture and head control after pulling the infant to sitting. Head control and posture were scored:

0—head passively hangs with no attempt to bring head upright; body slumps forward

1—head hangs down, but infant attempts to right head; spine and body slumped forward

2—head remains upright for several seconds with minimal movement

3—head remains upright with only several movements; upper spine is straightening up

4—head remains upright for three to four seconds and upper spine is straight

5—head is steady and upright; spine is straight but still needs some support

10. *Moro Reflex.* The examiner held the infant in the supine position. The reflex was elicited by a quick extension of the neck, allowing the head to drop into the examiner's hand. The response was described, and then objectively scored:

0—no response (within 30 seconds)

1—minimal abduction (less than 45 degrees) or extension (less than 45 degrees) of arms

2—minimal arm motion involving abduction or extension, or both, of greater than 45 degrees

3—full abduction or extension, or both, of the arms

4—immediate and full response to a short head drop

5—any handling elicits a Moro reflex

Prone

1. *Spontaneous Activity.* The infant was observed in the prone position for three minutes. Subjective observations regarding posture and movement were recorded.

2. *Head Lifting.* The examiner described the infant's attempt to clear his head from the supporting surface when placed in the prone position. The response was scored:

   0—no effort is made to clear the face

   1—a minimal effort involving visible contraction of neck muscles, but the face does not clear the surface

   2—the face is cleared several times for a few seconds

   3—sustained head lift for three to four seconds

   4—the head is cleared for ten seconds with any degree of clearance

   5—the head is upright with the face vertical to the supporting surface

3. *Tonic Labyrinthine Reflex.* The examiner first described the infant's posture when lying prone. The examiner then placed a hand beneath the infant's forehead and passively extended the head. The amount of resistance to passive motion was graded using the same scale as for the tonic labyrinthine reflex in the supine position.

4. *Galant's Reflex.* With the infant in the prone position, the examiner firmly stroked the paravertebral muscles in a cephalocaudal direction from approximately midthoracic area to low lumbar area. The response was scored:

   0—no response

   1—slight movement of spine and wrinkling of skin after repeated stimulation

   2—slight movement of spine to each stimulus

   3—obvious full spine incurvation with each stimulus

   4—obvious full trunk incurvation sustained for three seconds

5. *Ventral Suspension.* The examiner picked up the infant from the prone position, supporting the baby with both hands about the thorax. The posture the infant assumed was described and graded:

   0—no attempt to raise head

   1—several unsuccessful efforts to raise the head and neck; body mostly flexed over examiner's hands

   2—weak head raising successful but never attains the horizontal plane

3—head sustained in the horizontal plane for several seconds

4—head extended with retracted shoulders

5—head, shoulders, spine, and hips extended to horizontal

6—head, shoulders, spine, hips, and knees extended above the horizontal plane

Vertical

1. *Head Control When Held in Standing.* Subjective description.

2. *Placing Reaction of the Feet.* The examiner held the infant upright with both hands about the thorax. The dorsum of the foot was touched against the under edge of the table. The response was described and graded:

0—no response

1—stimulated leg flexed and then extended; foot is not placed

2—placing response, but difficult to elicit (requires repeated stimulation)

3—full placing response, easily elicited but placed briefly (only one or two stimulations needed)

4—full response, easily elicited and placed for ten seconds

6. The average examination time was ten minutes. Twenty minutes was the maximal time allotted for the examination, allowing time to calm the infant if he was crying or to stimulate him if he was asleep. If not completed within twenty minutes, the examination was discontinued and attempted at another time.

RESULTS

7. In general, alertness and reactiveness to stimuli increased with time, but fluctuations were noted in several scores on the days that hyperbilirubinemia was present, during time of body temperature instability, and when breast-feeding was initiated.

8. State differentiation evolved from a state of continual somnolence during the first two weeks of life, but especially the first days of life, to precisely defined states of sleep and wakefulness when the infant was about forty weeks of postmenstrual age. Concomitantly, N. M. became more active and responsive to stimuli.

Spontaneous Activity

9. Motor activity was almost totally suppressed during the first two days of life, then increased and fluctuated with changing medical conditions over the next two weeks, finally increasing steadily to attain

the maximal possible score (Table 1). Motor patterns noted during the early weeks of life included gyrating arm movements, bilateral reciprocal leg flexion and extension rolling to one side, hand-to-mouth activity, and head turning. Tremors were common. The motions of the premature infant were wide-ranging with more elbow, hip, and knee extension than are seen in the full-term infant. During the fourth week (38 weeks postmenstrual age), bridging (elevation of the hips in supine) was observed as well as reciprocal kicking and increased facial contact by the hands; although the activity level was high, there were fewer wildly gyrating limb movements than previously.

10.   In both supine and prone, flexion postures were assumed with increasing frequency, first in the legs and later in the arms as the infant matured. At no time, however, did the degree of hip, knee, or elbow flexion approach the degree of flexion seen in full-term neonates. In the prone position, a flexed posture with the arms flexed tightly against the chest was consistently observed. The hips were typically abducted and flexed, but occasionally assumed a relaxed extended posture. As N. M. became older, hip flexion increased and abduction decreased, causing the hips to elevate from the surface. They were, however, never adducted and flexed to the degree seen in full-term infants in the prone position.

Oral Reflexes

11.   Sucking and rooting activity were present immediately and increased gradually in strength and duration during the first week and one-half. The sucking score peaked on day 10 when breast feeding was initiated (Table). Both scores dropped in succeeding days and remained constant until the expected date of delivery when maximal ratings were again obtained. At eight weeks of age, the infant refused to suck when a nonnutritive stimulus was offered. Apparently, he was able to recognize the difference between breast and pacifier and, when hungry, reacted appropriately by refusing to suck a pacifier.

Muscle Tone

12.   The objective muscle tone ratings remained almost constant during the first eight weeks of life (Table). During the first days of life, little resistance to passive movement was encountered. Upon release of the limb, rebound occurred after a brief latency. The rebound in the early examinations was more brisk and consistent in the legs than in the arms. Resistance to displacement, especially to extension, progressed with maturation to such a degree that proximal stabilization was

Table 1. Ratings of developmental reflexes and motor patterns from day 1 to day 56 (approximately 42 weeks postmenstrual age) of postnatal life

Test Item	Item Rating[a]															
	Day 1	2	3	5[b]	6	7	8	9	10[c]	14	16	20	35	40	50	56
Supine																
Spontaneous activity	0	0	1	1	1	1	2	1	1	1	2	3	3	3	3	3
Sucking	2	2	2	1	3	3	3	3	4	3	3	3	4	4	3	3
Rooting	1	1	1	1	3	3	3	5	4	4	4	4	4	5	5	5
Palmar response	3	3	3	3	4	4	3	3	3	4	3	4	4	4	4	4
Tonic labyrinthine reflex	1	2	2	1	1	2	2	2	2	2	2	2	2	3	2	2
Muscle tone	2	2	2	2	2	2	2	2	2	2	2	2	2	2	2	2
Pull to sitting	1	1	1	1	2	2	1	2	3	3	2	4	4	4	4	4
Head control (sitting)	1	1	1	1	1	1	1	1	1	1	1	2	1	2	2	2
Moro reflex	2	3	3	2	3	4	4	4	3	4	4	4	4	4	4	4
Prone																
Head lifting	1	1	1	1	1	1	1	1	1	1	1	1	1	2	2	2
Tonic labyrinthine reflex	2	2	2	1	1	1	2	2	2	2	2	3	2	2	2	1
Galant's reflex	1	0	1	1	1	1	1	1	1	1	1	2	2	2	0	0
Ventral suspension	0	0	0	0	1	1	1	1	1	1	1	1	1	2	2	2
Vertical																
Placing reaction	0	0	0	0	1	1	1	0	1	1	1	2	2	3	3	3

[a] See text for scoring system.
[b] Hyperbilirubinemia diagnosed.
[c] Breast feeding initiated and body temperature fluctuations noted.

needed to obtain full extension of the limbs; nevertheless, full range of motion was always present in each joint, making it impossible for the infant to obtain a score above 2, despite the fact that resistance to displacement and the resulting rebound to the starting position became stronger over time.

Asymmetrical Tonic Neck Reflex

13.   Postural changes were first seen in the leg toward which the face was turned. The arms became consistently responsive during the second week of postnatal life. Trunk participation began at seven weeks of age (41 weeks postmenstrual age). The most consistently obtained response was elbow flexion on the occiput side. The reflex was never noted to be obligatory.

Head Control

14.   Head control during the pull-to-sitting test improved steadily until three weeks of age when righting the head was obtained after the first 45 degrees of trunk flexion (Table). This response remained static until the end of the study when the infant was two months old. In the sitting position, by the end of the first week, the baby was able to extend his head to the vertical, a position which seemed to facilitate ease of respiration. Attempts at head righting when supported in sitting became more effective with increasing age (Table). He began to rotate his head laterally during the third week of life at thirty-seven postmenstrual weeks and maintained his head in an oscillating, erect position for several seconds at six weeks of age.

15.   Head lifting in the prone position showed little change during the course of the study (Table). For the first month and a half, the infant made minimal efforts at neck extension involving visible contraction of neck muscles, but he was unable to clear his face from the supporting surface. At five weeks of age (approximately equal to term), he became able to clear his face repeatedly for a few seconds, a response which was still present at the end of the second month of life.

Ventral Suspension

16.   The ability of the infant to resist the force of gravity when supported about the thorax in ventral suspension improved gradually (Table). No response was noted during the first five days; head, trunk, and limbs conformed to the pull of gravity. From the end of the first week to the fifth week of age, the infant made several unsuccessful efforts to raise

192

his head during each test while the body remained flexed over the examiner's hands. At an age equivalent to term, the infant was able to raise his head successfully to a level slightly less than the horizontal plane, the best response obtained during the course of this study. The rest of the body never participated overtly in the reaction which begins at two to three months of age, according to Milani-Comparetti and Gidoni.[11] The knees and elbows remained extended; however, the trunk muscles showed a gradual increase in extensor tone as evidenced by decreased trunk curvature over the examiner's hand during suspension.

Moro Reflex

17.   The Moro reflex increased from an upper extremity response of slightly more than 45 degrees of shoulder abduction or elbow extension on day 2 to an immediate and full response to a short head drop by one week of age, a behavior which then remained stable (Table). The initial low postural tone of the infant was reflected in a large displacement of the arms when the Moro reflex was elicited. As flexor tone increased, the range of arm displacement decreased and the velocity of response increased. The range, however, remained greater than noted in a full-term infant with typical flexor hypertonicity.

Placing Reaction

18.   The placing reaction of the feet could not be elicited for the first five days (Table). It then appeared as a flexion-extension response of the leg following contact of the foot, but without placing. At three weeks of age, a full placing reaction could be elicited after repeated stimulation, and at five weeks of age the foot was placed for a few seconds after one or two stimulations.

19.   The tests of palmar grasp, tonic labyrinthine, and Galant's reflexes produced no reliable trends during the age period observed in this study, and the results of these tests will not be discussed further. The scores for these items are presented in the Table.

DISCUSSION

20.   Several major patterns of change emerged from the daily and weekly observations of this infant. These changes included differentiation of state, the influence of birth shock, and the quality and quantity of motor activity.

Birth shock was present during the first two days of life accounting for the minimal amount of spontaneous activity and a depressed sucking reflex. Beintema has reported a significant number of subjects with a depressed sucking reflex during the first four days of life,[10] and other studies have also attributed a depression in infant activity and responsiveness during the first few days of life to birthshock.[12,13] Escardo and de Coriat have reported a significant number of cases of birth shock resulting from anesthesia employed during labor.[12] A check of the mother's labor history revealed the use of anesthesia during labor.

21.　　As anticipated, the infant's activity level increased with age and with changes in physiological state. The level of spontaneous motor activity progressed from an initial level of minimal or no motor activity during the first weeks of life to an almost continually active infant during the final examination eight weeks later. The initial low level of motor activity was found in the presence of physiological instability, low muscle tone, and a state of somnolence.

22.　　In addition to increased quantity of motor activity, the overall quality of the infant's movements became more coordinated. In the first few weeks, arm and leg movements were bizarre, writhing, and often tremulous. As the infant matured, constraint of the wildly gyrating limbs occurred. Similar observations of mobility changes in premature infants have been noted by others.[2,3,14]

23.　　The first apparently intentional movements were noted in the oral area when the infant was able to differentiate nutritive from non-nutritive objects he was offered to suck. This behavior is acknowledged by Piaget as one of the infant's first intelligent acts, developed by repeated contacts with objects associated with either food or non-nutritive stimulation.[15] Sucking of the hand is used in self-comforting according to Brazelton,[16] but Burpee[17] has reported that premature infants from birth to forty weeks postmenstrual age appear to exhibit hand-mouth behaviors infrequently compared to full-term neonates.

24.　　The subjective descriptions and the objective scores for the selected test items appeared to reflect accurately the premature infant's motor development, as subjectively described by Saint-Anne Dargassies.[2,3] More specifically, the descriptions and scores document the caudocephalic development of muscle tone and its influence on motor development. The premature infant's muscle tone during the first days and weeks of life is essentially flaccid. The more premature the infant, the more flaccid he appears.[2,3] Correspondingly, little or no spontaneous activity accompanies the global hypotonia of the premature infant of twenty-eight to thirty weeks gestation. As the infant matures, his muscle tone develops progressively in a caudocephalic direction. Flexor muscle tone initially dominates in the legs, as was seen in N.M., and is observed in handling of the infant, in the quality of spontaneous movements, and in the resting postures of the infant, such as that produced by the asymmetrical tonic neck reflex. Eventually the flexor tone influence plateaus; however, previous to this flexor plateau, the development of extensor tone is occurring, resulting in active extension of the legs and, later, of the trunk when placed in standing, followed by decreased hip flexion in prone and initial attempts at neck extension. Eventually equilibration of these tonal influences becomes evident overtly in the attainment of a synergistic motor skill such as head control in sitting.

25.   Consistent differences from the full-term infant in postures and muscle tone were observed in the premature infant from birth to an age equivalent to forty-two weeks postmenstrual age. Not only is the muscle tone of the thirty-four- to thirty-five-week premature infant initially low and asymmetrically distributed between arms and legs, but the degree of flexor hypertonicity noted in the full-term neonate is never achieved.[2,3] The full-term neonate moves less than the premature infant, his ranges of movement being restricted by flexor hypertonicity. The premature infant, in contrast, has full range of motion into extension; resting postures feature less flexion and adduction of the hips than seen in the full-term infant; and stimulation of the Moro reflex results in wide opening of the arms.

26.   The apparent low flexor muscle tonicity in the premature infant may be caused by the early influence of gravity exerted on the postural, extensor musculature resulting in strong extensor muscles relative to flexor muscles. (The infant in utero, by contrast, is surrounded by amniotic fluid so that the extensor muscles are not subjected to an equivalent gravitational stretch, and he is experiencing an increasing amount of mechanical compression as parturition approaches.[18]) The flexor muscles of the premature are not *without* tone after the initial period of hypotonia. They are merely opposed by relatively stronger extensor muscles; thus, at term-equivalent age, the premature infant is able to initiate head righting when pulled to sitting from supine and successfully maintains an erect head for a few seconds in sitting, while the full-term neonate exhibits complete head lag when pulled up and makes only weak attempts at neck extension when held erect.[14] Early development of head control and of neck muscle cocontraction, therefore, appears to be facilitated by early experience.

27.   Unfortunately, the rating scale chosen to assess muscle tone, response to *passive* limb displacement, was not valid for the premature infant. The scale did not reflect early asymmetry between arms and legs, failed to measure all of the muscle tone changes which occurred, and showed almost no variance despite changes in posture

195

and movement observed during spontaneous activity and testing procedures.

28.   Observations of resistance to passive stretch do not appear useful in predicting the quality of performance of functional activities involving coordination of mobility and postural stability with adequate force, velocity, and sequence of muscle activation. Attempts to improve early recognition of central nervous system pathology must include development of a satisfactory quantitative assessment of postural tone since the authors have subjectively observed that muscle tone abnormalities, particularly in the legs, are often observed before retarded motor development or abnormal movement patterns are recognized in evaluation of the premature infant. In addition, clarification of the caudocephalic direction of muscle tone development is needed. Clearly, tonicity is present in the muscles of mastication before it becomes apparent more caudally, and sucking is a relatively mature skill even before birth. The actual timing of the appearance of tonicity in individual muscle groups remains to be described adequately.

29.   The Rosenblith Neonatal Behavioral Assessment Scale contains a comprehensive measure of muscle tone in which a rating is derived from several items, including resting posture, passive limb displacement, degree of trembling, and quality of resisted movement.[19] This scale may find increasing use as the test becomes more widely known and validated. Another approach to evaluation of muscle tone in infants might be use of the tonic vibration reflex to examine motoneuron excitability indirectly, [20-23] since the quality of tonic reflexes may have more significance than the phasic reflexes in the prediction of postural control abnormalities.

30.   The purpose of performing this clinical study was to enhance our understanding of neuromuscular development in the premature infant, especially in those areas in which it differs from that of the term infant. While evaluation of one infant is not sufficient for establishing developmental norms, it has assisted us in appreciating the quality of movement patterns in premature infants and comparing them with the patterns observed in full-term infants. This information is vital for physical therapists who evaluate high risk infants in the first months of life in order to avoid false identification of cerebral dysfunction. Large ranges of movement, trembling, relatively dominant extensor tone, and presence of asymmetrical tonic neck reflex effects on muscle tone in the legs are normal findings in the premature infant in the early weeks of postnatal life and, unless they persist, should not be interpreted as abnormal symptoms.

ACKNOWLEDGMENTS

Appreciation is expressed to the staff of the premature nursery at North Carolina Memorial Hospital, especially Ernest N. Kraybill, M.D., and Martha G. Russell, R.N., and to the parents of N.M. for their cooperation and support of this project.

REFERENCES

1. Michaelis, R., et al.: Activity states in premature and term infants. Psychobiol. 6:209, 1973.
2. Saint-Anne Dargassies, S.: The Development of the Nervous System in the Foetus. Monograph available from the author, centre neonatal de l'Association Claude Bernard, 123 Boulevard de Port-Royal, 75014 Paris, France. Switzerland, Nestle.
3. Saint-Anne Dargassies, S.: Neurological maturation of the premature infant of 28 to 41 weeks gestational age. In Faulkner, F. (ed.): *Human Development.* W. B. Saunders Company, Philadelphia, 1966.
4. Apgar, V.: The newborn (Apgar) scoring system. Pediatr. Clin. North Am 13:645, 1966.
5. Meadow, R.: Phototherapy and hyperbilirubinemia. Dev. Med. Child. Neurol. 12:802, 1970.
6. Prechtl, H., and Beintema, D. J.: The Neurological Examination of the Full Term Newborn Infant. Little Club Clinics in Developmental Medicine, no. 12. London, National Spastics Society, 1964.
7. André-Thomas, et al.: The Neurological Examination of the Infant. Little Club Clinics in Developmental Medicine, no 1. London, National Spastics Society, 1960.
8. Kraybill, E. N.: Personal communication, 1973.
9. Hutt, S. J., et al.: Psychophysiological Studies in Newborn Infants. In Lipsitt, L. P., and Reese, H. W. (eds.): Advances in Child Development and Behavior, vol 4. Academic Press, New York, 1969, pp. 128–172.
10. Beintema, D. J.: A Neurological Study of Newborn Infants. Little Club Clinics in Developmental Medicine, no 28. London, National Spastics Society, 1968.
11. Milani-Comparetti, G., and Gidoni, E. A.: Routine developmental examination in normal and retarded children. Dev. Med. Child. Neurol. 9:631, 1967.
12. Escardó, F., and de Coriat, L. F.: Development of postural and tonic patterns in the newborn infant. Pediatr. Clin. North. Am. 7:511, 1960.
13. Yang, D. C.: Neurologic status of newborn infants on first and third day of life. Neurology 12:72, 1962.
14. Illingworth, R. S.: The Development of the Infant and Young Child: Normal and Abnormal, ed. 5. The Williams & Wilkins Company, Baltimore, 1972.
15. Piaget, J.: The Origins of Intelligence in Children. International Universities Press, New York, 1952.
16. Brazelton, T. B.: Neonatal Behavioral Assessment Scale. Little Club Clinics in Development Medicine, no. 50. J. B. Lippincott Company, Philadelphia, 1973.
17. Burpee, B.: Hand-mouth Behaviors of Premature and Full Term Infants. Unpublished research, University of North Carolina at Chapel Hill, Chapel Hill, N.C., 1974.
18. Moore, K. L.: The Developing Human: Clinically Oriented Embryology. W. B. Saunders Company, Philadelphia, 1973.
19. Rosenblith, J. F.: Manual for Behavioral Examination of the Neonate, Modified by Judy F. Rosenblith (unpublished) from Graham, F. K.: Behavioral differences be-

tween normal and traumatized newborns: 1. The test procedures. Psychol. Monogr. 70:6, (no. 427), 1956. Manual available from author: Institute for Research in the Health Sciences, Brown University, Providence, RI.

20. Arcangel, C. D., et al.: The Achilles tendon reflex and the H-response during and after tendon vibration. Phys. Ther. 51:889, 1971.
21. Johnston, R. M., et al.: Mechanical vibration of skeletal muscles. Phys. Ther. 50:499, 1970.
22. Bishop, B.: Vibratory stimulation: Part I. Neurophysiology of motor responses evoked by vibratory stimulation. Phys. Ther. 54:1273, 1974.
23. Bishop, B.: Vibratory stimulation: Part II. Vibratory stimulation as an evaluation tool. Phys. Ther. 55:28, 1975.

BREATHING EXERCISES FOR CHILDREN WITH PSEUDOHYPERTROPHIC MUSCULAR DYSTROPHY*

Carolyn R. Houser, M.A., and Donna M. Johnson, M.A.

A controlled clinical trial designed to evaluate the effects of breathing exercises on the pulmonary function of a group of children with pseudohypertrophic muscular dystrophy is described. The rationale for the selection of the specific breathing exercises is discussed, and pretreatment and post-treatment results of standardized pulmonary function testing are reported.

1. The ultimate consequence of pseudohypertrophic muscular dystrophy is predominantly attributed to some variety of cardiorespiratory insufficiency or complicating respiratory infection.[1-4] Despite such widespread consistency in reporting, respiratory function during the course of the disease has seldom been studied. In the isolated instances where such investigation had been attempted, concurrence in the pulmonary disabilities was reported. Most commonly cited were significantly reduced vital capacity, maximal voluntary ventilation, and forced expiratory ability.[5-8] Clinical findings often in-

---

*Reprinted from *Physical Therapy* (51:751-759, 1971) with permission of the American Physical Therapy Association. Photographs have been omitted.

cluded inability to cough, chest wall restriction, and respiratory muscle weakness. [9-11]

2.   Efforts to improve pulmonary function, or at least retard its decline, are warranted for several reasons. The combination of inadequate defense against infection and reduced pulmonary reserves may predispose these patients to frequent and prolonged respiratory infections. [3, 12] These infections not only burden an already inadequate respiratory system, but also predispose to debilitating periods of immobility during the recovery process. Furthermore, surgical treatment of these patients is often limited by their questionable respiratory status. [8] The dystrophic child with inadequate respiratory reserve may be particularly liable to respiratory difficulty when exposed to the depressant action of general anesthesia. [13]

3.   Many of the pulmonary deficiencies present in these patients appear amenable to treatment with breathing exercises. Respiratory musculature is reported to be one of the last affected by the dystrophic process and, therefore, might be the most responsive to such a program. [1, 14, 15] Despite the frequent use of breathing exercises by physical therapists, their effectiveness with muscular dystrophy patients has seldom been evaluated through controlled study. This clinical study, therefore, was designed to test the hypothesis that a breathing exercise program would improve respiratory function, or retard its decline, in a group of children with pseudohypertrophic muscular dystrophy.

METHOD

4.   The sample consisted of fourteen wheelchair-bound boys with a diagnosis of pseudohypertrophic muscular dystrophy. The subjects ranged in age from eight to fifteen years and were receiving physical therapy while attending a school for handicapped children.

5.   An initial evaluation of the patients' pulmonary status included the following pulmonary function tests, administered by a registered inhalation therapist:

1. Forced Vital Capacity (FVC). The maximal amount of gas that can be forcefully expelled from the lungs following a maximal inspiration. [16]

2. Forced Expiratory Flow ($FEF_{25-75\%}$). The average flow rate during expulsion of the middle half of the forced vital capacity. [16, 17]

3. Maximal Voluntary Ventilation (MVV). The largest volume of air that can be moved into and out of the lungs in a given number of seconds. [18]

4. Peak Expiratory Flow Rate (PEFR). The highest flow rate sus-

tained for at least ten milliseconds during a single forced expiration.[19]

6. Each subject's breathing pattern, chest expansion, coughing ability, and abdominal and neck flexor strength were evaluated by the physical therapists conducting the study. A complete description of the testing methods and pretreatment findings are reported elsewhere.[6]

7. Following the initial tests, the subjects were ranked in order of performance on vital capacity determinations since this was considered the best single test of pulmonary reserve. Matched pairs were formed; each pair was then divided into experimental and control subjects by a table of random numbers. Table 1 permits comparison of the initial status of the treated and control subjects. The mean vital capacity of the control group was 67.5 percent of the predicted normal value, while the mean vital capacity of the experimental group was 65.5 percent. The mean ages of the experimental and control groups were 12.0 and 12.5 years, respectively.

8. The severity of the subjects' general physical involvement was evaluated by the eight-stage functional scale formulated by Swinyard, Deaver, and Greenspan.[20] The final, or eighth functional stage, which indicates the child must remain in bed, was modified according to Price to include subjects who could sit in a wheelchair with maximal support.[21] At the time of the study, all subjects were confined to wheelchairs and were performing at Functional Stage 5 or below. Table 2 describes the stages and indicates the similarity of functional abilities in the two groups.

Table 1. Comparison of age, functional ability, and initial forced vital capacity of matched pairs of treated and control subjects

| | | Treatment | | | Control | |
Pairs	Age	Functional Group[a]	FVC	Age	Functional Group	FVC
1	10–2	6	89.0%	10–7	6	94.0%
2	8–5	5	85.0%	8–5	5	82.0%
3	11–7	5	70.0%	11–5	6	77.0%
4	10–10	6	66.6%	12–10	5	66.6%
5	15–0	7	63.0%	15–0	7	63.0%
6	12–9	6	51.0%	13–11	7	52.0%
7	14–11	8	34.0%	15–6	8	38.0%
Mean	12–0	6.1	65.5%	12–5	6.2	67.5%

[a]Swinyard-Deaver Scale.

Table 2. Levels of functional ability of treated and control subjects

Functional Stage (Swinyard-Deaver Scale)	No. of Patients Treatment	Control
5. Independent in wheelchair activities and transfers	2	2
6. Propels wheelchair well but requires assistance for transferring	3	2
7. Propels wheelchair only short distances	1	2
8. Sits in wheelchair with support but cannot propel chair	1	1

9.   Though not a part of this investigation, all subjects received a similar program of therapeutic exercise and positioning during the course of the pulmonary function study. This program was designed to prevent further increases in the severity of hip and knee flexion contractures, promote circulation, and decrease the pain associated with prolonged periods of lower limb immobility.

10.   During the twelve-week study, the experimental group of seven subjects participated in a breathing exercise program five days per week. The program consisted of positive pressure breathing, six minutes daily. In addition, deep breathing exercises, assisted coughing, and games requiring forced expiration were employed three times per week.

11.   Positive pressure breathing was administered by means of a Bennett Pressure Breathing Therapy Unit* which assisted inflation of the lungs during inspiration. The flow-sensitive valve of the unit allowed the subject to initiate each breathing cycle by a slight inspiratory effort and, thus, control his own breathing rate. The child was asked to breathe slowly and deeply and to maintain the maximal inspiratory position briefly in order to ensure the most effective ventilation. An expiratory period longer than the inspiratory phase was encouraged to prevent hyperventilation and undue stress on the cardiac system. [22-24] During the first six weeks of treatment, a pressure of 10 centimeters of water was used. Throughout the second six weeks, the pressure was progressively increased to 18 centimeters of water. A monitoring spirometer attached to the unit allowed the child to observe the results of his inspiratory efforts and served as a means of reinforcement. Because of the subjects' weak abdominal musculature, snug-fitting ab-

---

*Bennett Respiration Products, Inc., 1639 11th St., Santa Monica, California 90404.

dominal binders were used to reduce expansion of the abdominal area
and encourage chest movement. [25]

12.   Deep breathing exercises were performed with the patients in a
semireclining position. A total of twelve deep inspirations was required during each session. A quick manual depression of the rib
margin at the beginning of inspiration was used to facilitate maximal
intercostal activity. Mild manual resistance was applied to both the intercostal and diaphragmatic areas to provide sensory cues for promoting the greatest function possible.

13.   The patients who could produce a functional cough practiced a coordinated cough pattern four to five times during the treatment session.
The remaining patients were assisted in coughing by use of abdominal
binders and the therapist's manual pressure over the abdomen. Each
effort was preceded by a maximal inspiration.

14.   Forced expiratory exercises were incorporated into games such as
blowing popcorn down a graduated track. Six maximal expiratory efforts were required, and each was preceded by a maximal inspiration.

15.   At the conclusion of the twelve-week breathing program, pulmonary
testing of the treated and control subjects was repeated.

RESULTS

16.   Comparison of measurements at the beginning and end of the treatment program are graphically reported in Figure 1 while the raw data
are presented in Table 3. Both experimental and control groups
showed decreased vital capacities over the twelve-week period. The
mean vital capacity decreased from 65.5 percent to 59.1 percent in the
treated group and from 67.5 percent to 58.9 percent in the control
group. The reduction was slightly less pronounced in the treated group
with a mean decline of 130 cubic centimeters (1,626 to 1,496 cc) as compared with 233 cubic centimeters (1,790 to 1,557 cc) in the control
group. While four of the seven treated subjects showed reductions, all
seven control subjects showed decreased vital capacities.

17.   Forced expiratory flow rates ($FEF_{25-75\%}$) also decreased for both
groups of patients, but, again, the mean decrease was less for the
treated group than for the control group. The mean percentage of
predicted values decreased from 94 percent to 90 percent for the
treated subjects while decreasing from 83 percent to 73 percent for the
control group. Of interest were the responses of the five subjects with
the lowest $FEF_{25-75\%}$ values, suggesting some form of airway obstruc-
tion. Two of these subjects were control subjects and showed further
decreases in their flow rates, while two of the three subjects in the
treated group showed increased flow rates.

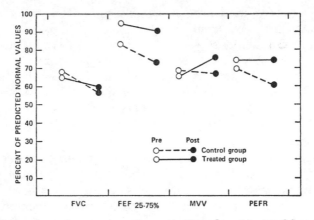

Figure 1. Comparison of mean scores on pretests and post-tests of four measures of pulmonary function in treated and control groups. (Fig. 3 in original article.)

18. On maximal voluntary ventilation determinations, a mean decrease of 1 percentage point was observed in the control group, while the experimental group showed a mean increase of 10 percentage points. The difference between the two groups was not significant at the .05 probability level when subjected to the Student's t test for correlated means. Six of the seven members of the treated group showed increased values while two members of the control group showed improvement.

19. A mean decrease was evident in both groups on peak expiratory flow rate. In terms of mean percent predicted values, the control group showed an average 9 percent decrease, while the experimental group demonstrated a 1 percent decrease. The difference between the two groups was not statistically significant.

20. No significant changes were noted in coughing ability, abdominal and neck flexor strength, breathing patterns, or chest expansion measurements.

DISCUSSION

21. The breathing exercises used in this study were selected after reviewing available literature and analyzing the pulmonary disabilities identified by initial testing. Deep breathing is normally a response to strenuous physical effort. In patients with muscular dystrophy, the generalized muscle weakness severely limits the level of physical activity. Thus, there may be need for eliciting maximal voluntary deep breaths to counteract the effects of respiratory muscle disuse.

Table 3. Summary of subjects' pretest and post-test findings on four measures of pulmonary function[a]

Percent of Predicted Values

Subjects	FVC			FEF$_{25-75\%}$			MVV			PERF		
	Pre	*Post*	*Change*	*Pre*	*Post*	*Change*	*Pre*	*Post*	*Change*	*Pre*	*Post*	*Change*
Control Group												
1	94.0	76.5	−17.5	112.0	116.0	+ 4.0	83.0	81.0	− 2.0	81.0	56.0	−25.0
2	82.0	77.0	− 5.0	78.0	83.0	+ 5.0	93.5	90.0	− 3.5	89.0	89.0	0.0
3	77.0	73.0	− 4.0	83.0	72.0	−10.0	56.0	55.0	− 1.0	59.0	55.0	− 4.0
4	66.6	55.5	−11.1	84.0	75.0	− 9.0	58.5	50.0	− 8.5	67.0	57.0	−10.0
5	63.0	58.0	− 5.0	95.0	73.0	−22.0	70.0	78.0	+ 8.0	65.0	56.0	− 9.0
6	52.0	42.0	−10.0	63.0	28.0	−35.0	43.0	51.0	+ 8.0	63.0	57.0	− 6.0
7	38.0	30.0	− 8.0	67.0	63.0	− 4.0	71.0	61.0	+10.0	61.0	51.0	−10.0
Means	67.5	58.9	− 8.6	83.1	72.9	−10.2	67.9	66.6	− 1.3	69.3	60.1	− 9.2
Treated Group												
1	89.0	61.0	−28.0	72.0	80.0	+ 8.0	49.5	54.0	+ 4.5	76.0	80.0	+ 4.0
2	85.0	74.0	− 9.0	105.0	114.0	+ 9.0	63.0	47.0	−16.0	69.0	60.0	−10.0
3	70.0	67.0	− 3.0	68.0	50.0	−18.0	60.0	75.0	+15.0	71.0	62.5	− 8.5
4	66.6	68.0	+ 1.4	140.0	116.0	−24.0	74.0	126.0	+52.0	79.0	78.0	− 1.0
5	63.0	56.6	− 6.4	130.0	121.0	− 9.0	98.0	104.0	+ 6.0	84.0	86.0	+ 2.0
6	51.0	53.0	+ 2.0	111.0	100.0	−11.0	60.0	64.0	+ 4.0	77.0	77.0	0.0
7	34.0	34.0	0.0	30.0	48.0	+18.0	55.0	59.0	+ 4.0	61.0	71.0	+10.0
Means	65.5	59.1	− 6.4	93.7	89.9	− 3.8	65.6	75.6	+10.0	73.9	73.5	+ 0.4

[a] *All data are recorded as the percentage of predicted normal values for subjects of the same age and height.*

205

22.   After noting the subnormal values on initial determinations of vital capacity and maximal voluntary ventilation, positive pressure breathing was incorporated into the treatment program for augmenting voluntary inspiratory volumes. The purpose of such augmentation was threefold. First, when weakness of the respiratory muscles prevents deep breathing, the assistance of positive pressure could provide better aeration of the alveoli and, thereby, reduce the tendency to develop atelectasis. Secondly, by providing a sensation of deep breathing, the assistance of positive pressure might also be useful for retraining the inspiratory muscles to their highest level of function. A third purpose of positive pressure breathing was to maintain compliance of the lungs and thorax.[26, 27] There is evidence that chest wall rigidity progressively increases in cases of thoracic muscle paralysis.[28] Lung compliance also appears to decrease when periodic deep breaths are absent.[29] These problems, resulting from weakness of the respiratory muscles, are further compounded when scoliosis produces structural changes in the rib cage and limits chest excursion.[30] Such spinal curvatures are frequently present in muscular dystrophy and were observed in six subjects participating in this study. If the musculature is allowed to shorten and fibrotic changes occur around the chest wall, increased demands will be placed on the weakening inspiratory muscles.[24] If flexibility of the rib cage could be maintained or increased by positive pressure breathing, less work would be required for maximal ventilation of the lungs.

23.   Nonfunctional coughs were noted in ten of the fourteen patients. This inability to cough might be attributed to several defects. Muscle testing revealed marked weakness of the abdominal musculature which would impair development of the increased intra-abdominal and intrathoracic pressures required for coughing. Furthermore, the reduced vital capacities evident from testing would suggest that the patients were unable to inspire a large enough volume of air for an adequate expulsive flow rate.

24.   Since coughing is vital for clearing the airways, efforts were directed toward strengthening and coordinating weakened cough mechanisms through practice and the addition of external manual assistance to increase intra-abdominal pressure. No subject with an ineffective cough was found to develop an effective cough during the twelve-week treatment program. Manual assistance, however, did appear to increase the forcefulness of the cough. It might prove beneficial to teach the family such methods of assisting coughing and to urge their application whenever the child's need to raise secretions becomes apparent.

25.   Only one study of the use of breathing exercises with muscular dystrophy patients was found in the literature. Seven subjects with

vital capacities below 75 percent of predicted normal participated in the study. Their ages ranged from seven to fourteen years. The investigator reported improved vital capacity values following institution of an intensive four-mouth rehabilitation program which included breathing exercises, but no data were included.[31]

26.   By contrast, in the present study a small decrease in vital capacity was observed over as short a period as twelve weeks in both the treated and control groups. Arce-Gomez and colleagues, and Hapke also report declining vital capacities in nontreated groups over nine-month and three-year periods, respectively.[5,7]

27.   Comparison of the changes in FVC and $FEF_{25-75\%}$ values for the control and treated groups suggests that a breathing program can help to retard the decline of pulmonary function. Maximal voluntary ventilation, however, was the only test where increased percent predicted values suggests the possibility of improved pulmonary function. Spirographic tracings indicate that such improvement was the result of greater endurance in five subjects and increased volumes in one subject.

28.   The fact that improvement in this small sample was not statistically significant at the .05 probability level does not preclude the possible effectiveness of the treatment in individual subjects. Improved function on the pulmonary tests was not limited to those subjects with the mildest physical and pulmonary involvement as might have been expected. Of the treated subjects that showed improvement, the greatest change was noted in one subject who showed moderate pulmonary and general physical involvement and in another who demonstrated severe physical disability and the lowest vital capacity of the fourteen subjects. The treated subjects demonstrated improvement on two and three of the four tests, respectively, while the two control subjects showed decreasing values on all tests (Table 4).

29.   The limited improvement observed in individual subjects over the

Table 4. Difference between pretreatment and post-treatment findings in two selected pairs of subjects (Pair 4—moderately involved; Pair 7—severely involved)

	FVC	MVV	$FEF_{25-75\%}$	PEFR
Pair 4				
Treated	+ 50 cc.	+49.3 1 pm	−24 1 pm	− 5 1 pm
Control	−300 cc.	− 7.2 1 pm	−13 1 pm	−35 1 pm
Pair 7				
Treated	− 25 cc.	+ 3.4 1 pm	+18 1 pm	+45 1 pm
Control	−270 cc.	− 7.2 1 pm	− 4 1 pm	−40 1 pm

short period of this study justifies a larger investigation involving long-term treatment and follow-up. Evaluation of each component of the program is also needed to prevent needless duplication and poor utilization of treatment time. Because of the varied response observed in the subjects, it appears vital that such treatment be accompanied by periodic, objective evaluation of individual responses to treatment. For children with progressive muscular dystrophy, a poor response might preclude or contraindicate further treatment in an intensive breathing program.

SUMMARY

30. A program of selected breathing exercises was administered to seven boys with pseudohypertrophic muscular dystrophy. The respiratory function of these subjects and their matched controls was evaluated by a series of respiratory and neuromuscular function tests. Comparison of the test results before and after a twelve-week experimental period revealed reduced values of both groups on determinations of vital capacity, forced expiratory flow rate, and peak expiratory flow rate. The treated group showed less decline than their controls. Mean values for maximal voluntary ventilation decreased in the control group while increasing in the experimental group. The differences in the two groups were not statistically significant in terms of these tests. A larger investigation is needed to support this study's suggestion that a program of breathing exercises may, in selected cases, retard the decline of respiratory function.

ACKNOWLEDGMENTS

Mrs. Wilma Bright, R.I.T., administered the pulmonary function tests.

Clinical Specialties, San Francisco, California, provided the positive pressure units for this study.

REFERENCES

1. Bourne, G.: Muscular Dystrophy in Man and Animals. Hafner Publishing Company, New York, 1963.
2. Dubowitz, V.: Muscular dystrophy and related disorders. Postgrad. Med. J. 41:332, 1965.
3. Gilroy, J., et al.: Cardiac and pulmonary complications in Duchenne's progressive muscular dystrophy. Circulation 27:484, 1963.
4. Walton, J. N.: The child with muscular dystrophy. Practitioner 192:478, 1964.
5. Arce-Gomez, E., et al.: Study of the cardiorespiratory function in patients with progressive muscular dystrophy. Angiology 15:407, 1964.

6. Burke, S. S., et al.: Respiratory aspects of pseudohypertrophic muscular dystrophy. Am. J. Dis. Child. 121:230, 1971.
7. Hapke, E. J.: Pulmonary function in progressive muscular dystrophy. In: Research in Muscular Dystrophy, Proceedings of the Fourth Symposium on Current Research in Muscular Dystrophy, edited by Members of the Research Committee of the Muscular Dystrophy Group. Pitman Medical Publishing Company, London, pp. 461–467.
8. Saheki, B., et al.: The studies on the pulmonary function of the patients of progressive muscular dystrophy. Iryo 21:794, 1967.
9. Gucker, T.: Muscular defects. Pediatr. Clin. North Am. 14:439, 1967.
10. Mullendore, J. M., and Stoudt, R.: Speech patterns in muscular dystrophic individuals. J. Speech Hear. Disord. 26:252, 1967.
11. Kenrick, M. M.: Certain aspects of managing patients with muscular dystrophy. South. Med. J. 58:996, 1965.
12. Dowben, R. M.: Seminar Int. 10:2, 1961.
13. Cobham, K. G.: Anesthesia for muscular dystrophy patients. Anesth. Analg. 43:22, 1964.
14. Magee, K.: The muscular dystrophies. Clin. Med. 69:1933, 1962.
15. Walton, J. N.: Progressive muscular dystrophy. Postgrad. Med. 35:102, 1964.
16. Boren, H. G., et al.: The Veterans Administration-Army cooperative study of pulmonary function, II. The lung volume and its subdivisions in normal men. Am. J. Med. 41:96, 1966.
17. Slonin, N. B.: Cardiopulmonary Laboratory Basic Methods and Calculations. Charles C Thomas, Springfield, Ill., 1967.
18. Motley, H.: Pathologic physiology of respiration. In Naclerio, E. A. (ed.): Bronchopulmonary Diseases—Basic Aspects, Diagnosis and Treatment. EA. Paul B. Hoeber, New York, 1957.
19. Wright, B. M., and McKerrow, C. B.: Maximum force expiratory flow rate as a measure of ventilatory capacity. Br. Med. J. 46:1041, 1959.
20. Swinyard, C. A., et al.: Gradients of functional ability of importance in rehabilitation of patients with progressive muscular and neuromuscular diseases. Arch. Phys. Med. 38:574, 1957.
21. Price, A.: Regression of Function in Pseudo-hypertrophic Muscular Dystrophy. American Occupational Therapy Association Monograph, No. 1. North Shore Publishing Company, Milwaukee, 1965.
22. Fairley, H. B.: Principles and practice of mechanical ventilation. Appl. Ther. 10:36, 1968.
23. Pace, W.: Pulmonary Physiology in Clinical Practice. F. A. Davis Company, Philadelphia, 1965.
24. Loehning, R., et al.: Intermittent positive pressure breathing therapy. In Safar, P. (ed.): Respiratory Therapy. F. A. Davis Company, Philadelphia, 1965.
25. Dail, C. W.: Respiratory aspects of rehabilitation in neuromuscular conditions. Arch. Phys. Med. 46:655, 1965.
26. Warren, A.: Mobilization of the chest wall. Phys. Ther. 48:582, 1968.
27. Whittenberger, J. L., and Ferris, B. G.: Impairment of the mechanics of respiration—paralytic conditions. In Gordon, B. L. (ed.): Cardiopulmonary Physiology. Grune and Stratton, New York, 1957.
28. Adkins, H.: Improvement of breathing ability in children with respiratory muscle paralysis. Phys. Ther. 48:577, 1968.
29. Bendixen, H. H., et al.: Pattern of ventilation in young adults. J. Appl. Physiol. 19:195, 1964.
30. Levine, D. B.: The influence of spinal deformities on chest function. In Hislop, H., and Sanger, J. (eds.): Chest Disorders in Children, Proceedings of a Symposium. American Physical Therapy Association, New York, 1968.
31. Hobermann, M.: Physical medicine and rehabilitation: Its value and limitations in progressive muscular dystrophy. Am. J. Phys. Med. 34:109, 1955.

TEMPORAL ADAPTATION: A CONCEPTUAL FRAMEWORK FOR OCCUPATIONAL THERAPY*

Gary Kielhofner

The concept of temporal adaptation was introduced into the field of occupational therapy early in its development; however, it has not been developed as part of the theoretical backing of the field. This paper re-introduces the theme and provides both a general perspective for the clinician in thinking about patients' temporal behavior and a preliminary framework for application. Temporal adaptation when applied in clinical practice should add a wider perspective to existing clinical interventions. It is proposed as a generically applicable theoretical perspective appropriate across all dysfunctional categories of patients. Two case histories are presented to demonstrate the application of the theoretical framework to intervention.

1.   In 1922, Adolf Meyer proposed a philosophy of practice for the newly formed profession of occupational therapy. He maintained that the key to successful application of occupational therapy would lie in an awakening to:

---

*Reprinted with permission of the American Occupational Therapy Association, Inc., from the *American Journal of Occupational Therapy* 31: 235–242, 1977.

> ... a full meaning of time as the biggest wonder and asset of our lives and the valuation of opportunity and performance as the greatest measure of time. . . . [1]

Eleanor Clarke Slagle pioneered the application of Meyer's proposal that occupational therapy should view patients within the context of time through the unfolding of their daily lives. She implemented a program of "habit training" based on the principle that the normal use of time in a purposeful daily routine would exert an organizing force on even the most regressed, unmedicated mentally ill patients.[2] Slagle intuitively recognized habit as a critical regulator of man's use of time and consequently as a significant component of his adaptation.

2. From Meyer and Slagle the profession received the proposition that in the richness of man's daily routines and his purposeful use of time, there was both health-maintaining and health-regenerating potential. Further, the way in which disabled individuals used and organized their time in daily life was revealed as a measure of their adaptiveness. Health was revealed in how patients functioned on a day-by-day, hour-by-hour basis. The temporal dimension in human adaptation was installed as a legitimate concern for occupational therapists. This temporal perspective gave to occupational therapy a special caretaker position for patients' activities of daily living.

3. However, occupational therapy practice has subsequently evolved away from a concern for patients' temporal functioning.[3] The full appreciation of the meaning of time, which Meyer so strongly advocated, never came to pass in occupational therapy. Consequently, the broad humanistic theme of activities of daily living suffered a substantial loss of content. Presently, the concept of activities of daily living conveys little more than a checklist for self-care.[4]

4. At a time when occupational therapy must face the reality of its "derailment," as Shannon suggests in his paper, it is imperative that the profession scrutinize its underpinnings and carefully examine its philosophy and practice for critical concepts that have been lost. The task that lies before the profession is to reclaim and revitalize those elements which made occupational therapy such a viable and energizing idea for the founders and early leaders of the profession.

5. The theme of temporal adaptation is a valuable scheme for practice and should be reintroduced to occupational therapy. Therefore, this paper first provides support for temporal functioning as a useful conceptual base from which human adaptation and dysfunction of the disabled can be better understood. Second, it proposes a temporal conceptual framework that serves as a background from which to generate evaluations and interventions.

6.   The elderly person whose abundant leisure has become painful monotony, the physically disabled person whose self-care has been expanded into a long and tedious procedure, the psychiatric patient whose personal helplessness makes the future an unwelcome burden, and the mentally subnormal person for whom the string of events in time seems a jumble . . . each represent a special difficulty in temporal adaptation. Although occupational therapists are thoroughly acquainted with such temporal problems, the systematic application of clinical intervention aimed at temporal dysfunction is not formally or consistently part of the clinician's treatment. In order to reintroduce temporal adaptation to clinical practice, this section provides a general theoretical overview. *Temporal adaptation* serves in this paper as a descriptive term for integration of an entire spectrum of activities, the organization of which supports health on an ongoing daily life basis. *Temporal dysfunction* will refer to problems that arise in this daily life organization. Temporal adaptation and dysfunction represent descriptive terms for talking about complex daily activity from the specific but universal dimension of time.

7.   *Time.* Time is the inescapable boundary for human existence and activity. Hall describes it as the "unconscious determinant or frame upon which everything else is built,"[5] and Henry states that for man time is a universal dimension, guiding and structuring his experience and his activity.[6] Human adaptation is inextricably bound up in the conscious experience of time. Man's conscious placement in time is a function of the capacity to symbolize internally that which is perceived externally.[7] Each man bears a complex symbolic model or image of himself located in time.[8] His initial awareness of time results from the experience of change in the self and the environment.[9] The model or image of external temporal reality is generated and continuously reorganized through the accumulated experience of changing events.

8.   Armed with temporal consciousness, man is a supreme actor in time. Not only is he aware of changing events, but he is likewise conscious of the fact that he can have some effect on that course of events. The perception of the self as a cause comes from experiencing the results of one's own actions in time.[10] Man's awareness of time, the awareness of his causative ability, and its potential for consequences are interrelated phenomena. The human condition is transformed by the awareness of the individual that he or she has acted, is acting, and will continue to act. Man's awareness of time makes possible this conti-

nuity of experience that transforms the nature of his adaptation. In John Dewey's words:

9.   Man differs from the lower animals because he preserves his past experiences . . . . With the animals, an experience perishes as it happens and each new doing or suffering stands alone. But man lives in a world where each occurrence is charged with echoes and reminiscences of what has gone before, where each event is a reminder of other things. Hence he lives not, like the beasts of the field, in a world of merely physical things, but in a world of signs and symbols. [11]

10.   Although overt experiences occur as disconnected and episodic events, the inner symbolic experience is an uninterrupted flow in which past and future are orienting reference points for human adaptation. Man draws upon his past experiences as an information source for future action. He projects himself into the future, planning events, and setting goals that may not be realized for days, months, or even years. Through imagination, he can test alternative courses of action and contemplate their consequences. [7] Once placed consciously in time, the human organism adapts through purposeful action. Man adapts through awareness of his own agenthood and placement in time that makes possible the conscious planning of action. Action and time are concomitant components of the human experience linked to purpose through hindsight and foresight.

THE CONCEPTUAL FRAMEWORK

11.   The concepts of temporal adaptation can be put into operation through a conceptual framework designed to generate strategies of evaluation and treatment in occupational therapy. A preliminary framework was constructed as a series of propositions about temporal adaptation. The first four concern external factors and learning that influence temporal experience and activity. Propositions five and six concern the internal organization of temporal behavior. The seventh proposition concerns pathologies or dysfunctions of time.

12.   *Proposition 1: Each person bears a temporal frame of reference that is culturally constituted.* Individuals carry an image of their placement in time that is a unique product of their culture. [12] Their temporal frame of reference is maintained and transmitted within the culture in the form of norms and values and contains the basic notion and valuation of time. [13]

213

13.   In American society the notion of time is that of a straight line or path extending into the future. Time is experienced as a "supersensible medium or container, as a stream of infinitely extended warp upon which the woof of human happenings is woven.... "[14] It is sectioned off and takes on the nature of enclosed or finite space, the segments of which are to be filled with activity.[12, 13] This notion of time is exhibited in the American habit of scheduling events. Random behavior that lacks a pattern of organization is not functional in the mainstream of American society.[6] The American culture values time as a commodity; it can be bought, sold, saved, or wasted.[13] This sense of time is captured in the phrase *"time is money"* and, understandably, wasting time has a strong negative connotation in the culture.

14.   Although the orderly, punctual life of Americans is not an innate feature of human existence, it is largely considered a fact of nature. This notion and valuation of time is the framework of the culture that sets boundaries for competent action in daily life. In order to adapt to the society the individual must to some degree internalize and order behavior according to the culture's temporal frame of reference.

15.   *Proposition 2: A unique temporal frame of reference is accumulated through learning and socializing experiences that begin in childhood.* Although the basic ability to perceive time is a cognitive developmental phenomenon, the particular culture frame of reference is a product of socialization.[6] The transmission of the temporal frame of reference has been classified by Hall into three levels of socialization or learning: technical, informal, and formal.[13]

16.   The technical learning of time occurs in a didactic framework, as when a child is taught to tell time and to comprehend the division of seconds, minutes, and hours. Informal time is learned through imitation of role models and the learning comprises activities and mannerisms that are so much a part of daily life that they are performed almost unconsciously. An example of informal time is knowing that being 5 minutes late for an appointment is acceptable, whereas 20 minutes is not. Formal learning is taught by precept and admonition, and concerns traditions and values transmitted through the expectations and prohibitions of each culture. As an example, the prohibition of wasting time is passed on in American culture as an important value.

17.   From this teaching, modeling, precept, and admonition, children's socialization is accomplished through the internalization of a complex temporal frame of reference. It is within the family that children first learn to organize time under this framework toward fulfillment of a social role. The role of children or siblings within the family bears with it a whole set of activities ordered in time. Learning to be on time for

meals, to do chores when assigned, to habitually care for themselves, and to periodically clean their rooms are all part of the complex schema children must incorporate. Learning temporal organization, which occurs within the family, generalizes to other roles children must take on later. Children not only know a particular set of behaviors ordered in time, but more importantly, also learn to organize activity in time.

18.   In addition to learning how and when to behave, children learn a complex set of temporal expectations; Toffler gives the following poignant description.

19.   From infancy on the child learns, for example, that when Daddy

> . . . leaves for work in the morning, it means that he will not return for many hours . . . . The child soon learns that "mealtime" is neither a one-minute nor a five-hour affair, but that it ordinarily lasts from fifteen minutes to an hour. He learns that going to a movie lasts two to four hours, but that a visit with the pediatrician seldom lasts more than one. He learns that the school day ordinarily lasts six hours. He learns that a relationship with a teacher ordinarily extends over a school year, but that his relationship with his grandparents is supposed to be of much longer duration. Indeed some relationships are supposed to last a lifetime. [15]

Where the household temporal patterns are chaotic, children's learning of the temporal frame of reference may be maladaptive. [6] Consequently, competent participation in the culture may be hindered as they falter in organizing time to respond to other successive social institutions, such as school and the job setting.

20.   *Proposition 3: There is a natural temporal order to daily living organized around the life-space activities of self-maintenance, work, and play.* Adolph Meyer pointed out that there is a natural rhythm in the organization of daily life around life spaces. [1] These life spaces are assigned to activities that represent a social order, determining appropriate times for role behavior. Reilly conceptualized daily living as divided into life spaces of existence, subsistence, and discretionary time. [16] Existence is that time spent for eating, sleeping, personal hygiene, and other aspects of self-maintenance; subsistence is the life space devoted to working for an income; and discretionary time is that life space reserved for recreation and leisure. Recreation and leisure comprise dual aspects of play in adult life. Recreation is the period of time when man is made ready for the next cycle of work through relaxation. Leisure is earned time made possible by satisfying performance of work.

215

21. Health consists of the proper balance of the life spaces that is both satisfying to individuals and appropriate for their roles within society. Balance refers to more than just so much work, play, and rest. Rather, balance recognizes an interdependence of these life spaces and their relationship to both internal values, interests, and goals, and external demands of the environment. It is the interrelated balance of self-maintenance, work, and play that comprises health.

22. While homeostasis is used to describe the biological health of the organism, a broader concept of balance in daily life describes the conditions for psychosocial health of the human organism. Occupational therapists are in a position to make critical statements about the health of their patients from both interrelated dimensions of homeostasis and balance. Far from being limited to the idea of self-care, activities of daily living refer to man's total state of health, which depends on both biological and psychosocial factors.

23. *Proposition 4: Society requires its members to organize their use of time according to ascribed social roles.* While cultural norms and values provide a contextual framework for man's use of time, his individual daily pattern must be organized around his occupational roles.[17] Heard expands on this theme of role behavior in her paper. The sum total of man's activity within his life spaces has been referred to as occupational behavior.[18] Life spaces are filled according to the occupational roles to which they are assigned. Within the daily routine, an individual's life spaces may be divided between several occupational roles such as the father, worker, and community volunteer. Adaptation requires individuals to use their time in a manner that supports their roles. The student must organize time for attendance at classes and homework, the worker for the job schedule, and the retiree for effective and satisfying use of leisure time.

24. The organization of time around one's roles is not a static skill. Occupational roles change and overlap; each individual passes through a succession of roles in a lifetime.[19] Taking on a new role requires a new strategy for organizing one's time. When role change is abruptly forced upon an individual through an incurred disability, developing new temporal skills is a critical factor in adapting to the disability.

25. *Proposition 5: An individual's use of time is a function of internalized values, interests, and goals.* Values are commitments to action that organize an individual's use of time by establishing an internal order of what comes first and how much time will be allotted to various activities.[20] An individual's values set priorities of actions, and their consequences create a personal valence that is ultimately translated into a life style. Values serve an important function in the choice an individual makes to take on various roles. Although values reflect more

serious commitments, interests also guide the commitment process. They are states of readiness for choices and action.[21] Interests sustain action and serve thereby to maintain commitments over time. Like values, interests prioritize activities and lend organization to temporal behavior.

26.   Goals represent strategies toward the fulfillment of values and interests. Values and interests yield automatic goal-setting and consequent adjustment and organization of daily patterns of time use. This process occurs at various levels of awareness and is necessary for ordering daily life. The individual who has no goals or has difficulty setting goals cannot organize daily life to use existing skills effectively and will, consequently, feel frustrated or helpless.[22,23] Further, an individual must be able to identify and execute appropriate actions for goal-attainment. Problems arise when an individual cannot identify and carry out in proper sequence those activities that lead to successful goal achievement.[23,24] Robinson expands this notion, sequencing action in time, in her paper on rules.

27.   *Proposition 6: Habits are the basic structures by which daily behavior is ordered in time and psychosocial health is maintained.* While habits are traditionally thought of in terms of vices and virtues, they extend a more subtle and profound influence on daily temporal functioning. All that is familiar, routine, and predictable in daily life bears a relationship to habit. Without habit structure, an individual's daily life would be a chaotic series of disjointed events.

28.   Habits are instantaneous, automatic choices of action made throughout the day.[3] Although organized into unconscious routines, they are the products of once conscious choices made until they become automatic.[3] Habits reflect actions related to values and interests cemented over time in daily patterns. Further, habits provide a crucial service to adaptation by organizing temporal behavior to meet societal requirements for competence. Consequently, habits perform an important role in assuring that skills are used in an adaptive manner. Skills must not only be present, but also organized into a daily routine.

29.   *Proposition 7: Temporal dysfunction may exist in relationship to categories of pathology.* Temporal dysfunction may occur as an integral part of some mental illness or as a consequence of imposed physical disability.

30.   When viewing individuals from the perspective of temporal adaptation, it becomes obvious that strategies for intervention cannot begin and end with the physical, mental, or emotional pathology. Each may be integrally related to a broader and often more difficult set of problems in the person's temporal adaptation.

31. Persons who are so disoriented in time that they cannot give the day, month, or year are readily suspected of being afflicted with amentia, senility, or some psychotic disorder.[12] Actual distortions of the perception of time have been shown to occur in some cases of mental illness.[9] Further, when individuals cannot organize their time toward fulfillment of their social roles, they may become candidates for psychiatric care.[24] Disorganization of time is associated with the subjective sense of helplessness and incompetence seen in mental illness.

32. Disorganization of temporal adaptation may also be identified in the reaction of an individual to residual physical disabilities. Maintaining a pace of life comparable to individuals without disability may be impossible for some persons whose motor performance is dysfunctional. The impact of sudden disability often imposes tremendous distortions of daily life spaces by increasing the amount of time required for routine activities. Further, where one or more roles change or end as a result of acquired physical disability, the individual may be unable to find new meaningful activities and roles to fill the life-spaces formerly occupied by old ones.

IMPLEMENTATION

33. Propositions were formulated as a guiding framework for incorporating temporal adaptation into clinical evaluation and treatment. The clinician may use the framework for integrating clinical data with points raised in the propositions. The framework gives the clinician another dimension for viewing patient problems and for generating and interpreting data. It thereby serves as a basis for developing new treatment strategies. Three principles should be adhered to in applying the conceptual framework to evaluation. First, data should be collected on several variables contained in the propositions. Relevant data include the patient's values, interests, goals, balance of play and work, habit structure, and temporal frame of reference. Second, the evaluation should take into consideration internal constraints on time as revealed in the nature of the patient's physical, mental, or emotional disability. Third, the evaluation should also consider the external factors influencing time use: the patient's roles, family expectations, cultural background, and the demands of time and physical space that affect the patient's daily living.

34. Treatment intervention will be based on the particular pattern of temporal dysfunction revealed by the evaluation. As data is interrelated and considered in light of the conceptual framework, dysfunctional patterns should become evident. For example, one patient's chaotic day may be a reflection of a lack of ability to prioritize in-

terests and to set goals. Without the ability to set priorities and goals, the patient cannot generate habits for a normal, satisfactory daily routine. By using the conceptual framework of temporal adaptation, the clinician should be able to formulate a more comprehensive treatment plan.

CASE EXAMPLES

35. Two case histories, together with examples of clinical interventions that follow the principles above, are presented to serve as examples of how the temporal adaptation framework can be applied. Treatments described speak only to the temporal framework and assume the inclusion of other traditional occupational therapy interventions.

Case H.B.

36. H.B. is a 24-year-old, single male psychiatric patient. When admitted to the hospital, his presenting problems included depression and chronic repeated failures in work settings. H.B. graduated from college with a degree in music with plans to re-enter college for graduate study in musicology. He not only has definite skills as a musician but has also demonstrated a strong commitment by voluntarily organizing a teenage choir in a local church.

37. However, H.B. has not managed during the last three years to hold down a steady job and save enough money to re-enter college. His recent occupational history includes such jobs as working in an electrical shop repairing fans, driving a school bus, and doing maintenance work in apartment complexes. H.B. was fired from each of these jobs because of his inability to concentrate on the work. He found the jobs uninteresting and had difficulty applying himself. He attempted to save money toward college, but used up his savings during periods of unemployment between jobs.

38. H.B. describes his daily life as highly variable and without routine. He has been unable to maintain any schedule and often finds himself late for work and appointments. Further, social activities have taken up a large part of his schedule so that he is negligent in doing many basic self-maintenance tasks. His housekeeping recently became so disorganized that he was evicted from his apartment. H.B. perceives his daily life as chaotic and complains that "there is so little time with so much to do, that I often get stuck on things and never get around to what I set out to do." He feels helpless and depressed since he is not close to his goal of re-entering college and does not feel he is progressing toward it. At this point his response to this subjective state is to

219

become inactive. He is without a job and recently does not even pursue his interests in music on a leisure basis.

29.   When considered in light of the conceptual framework, H.B.'s temporal dysfunction can be outlined as follows. H.B. has internalized values and goals. He considers further education important and realistically has chosen an area of study within his capacities. His temporal dysfunction lies in the areas of: (a) identifying and pursuing reasonable short-term objectives that will bring him closer to his overall goal; (b) maintaining a satisfying daily schedule that would balance activities of work, play, and self-maintenance; and (c) organizing his time around present necessary role of being a worker. The temporal dysfunction that has eroded his competence in several areas augments his feelings of depression and helplessness.

40.   Recommendations for treatment should include: (1) assisting H.B. in identifying how his present worker role will lead to the eventual goal of re-entering college and developing a strategy that balances his interest in music with the necessity of working on a daily basis; (2) practice in formulating a basic, balanced daily routine and adhering to it consistently; and (3) making beginning steps toward his overall goal, by gathering information on graduate programs in music, their requirements, and possible scholarships. By subdividing each of these goals into subroutines such as finding a new job or ways of pursuing his interest in music on a leisure basis, he may be able to overcome the vicious cycle of daily life incompetence, helplessness, and depression. Treatment would occur in graded steps toward the eventual reconstruction of daily living skills.

Case T.J.

41.   T.J. is a 17-year-old male who sustained a spinal cord injury in an automobile accident. Five months after the injury, T.J., a paraplegic, remains depressed and withdrawn. When approached about his depressed state, T.J. responds that his life-plans have been destroyed. Prior to his injury he was an excellent athlete with a promise of an athletic scholarship to a university. Beyond his college training, T.J. had hoped to become a high school coach. Further, T.J. points out that he is now forced to spend days in bed or a wheelchair, whereas formerly he was active in a variety of intramural and varsity sports. He describes the present as boring and sees little prospect for change in the future. Also data from his family points out that T.J.'s former positive self-image revolved around his physical appearance and athletic prowess; he now views himself as an invalid.

42.   In T.J.'s case it should be noted that: (a) his former values and in-

220

terests focused on activities he can no longer engage in or he must learn to participate in with some modifications; (b) his self-image and prospects for the future revolved around skills and capacities no longer intact; (c) his former daily routine revolved around hs athletic role. In summary, those values and habits that formerly maintained a satisfying daily routine and those skills and goals which made the future desirable are no longer intact.

48.   T.J.'s treatment under the framework of temporal adaptation would focus on the following sequence of treatment strategies: (1) reconstruction of the self-image through successful experiences in areas related to his past interests; (2) exploration of new activities to develop interests (in the clinic and his own community); (3) reconstruction of his daily routine, which will have to accommodate different life spaces—such as the expanded space necessary for self-care and personal hygiene; and (4) refocusing on his career goals so that a viable and acceptable objective could at least be tentatively pursued.

CONCLUSION

44.   Temporal adaptation was identified as an early theme in occupational therapy that has been dropped out of clinical practice. The concept of temporal adaptation was reintroduced and formulated in a preliminary framework for clinical intervention. Temporal adaptation serves as a conceptual schema to broaden the clinician's current perspective and repertoire of skills and, as such, does not replace traditional therapeutic efforts but expands them into a more comprehensive framework. Temporal adaptation is a rich conceptual schema for occupational therapy because it speaks to a class of dysfunction found in the entire range of patients seen by occupational therapists.

ACKNOWLEDGMENTS

This article is based in part upon material submitted in partial fulfillment of the requirements for the Master of Arts Degree, University of Southern California, Los Angeles. Partial financial support for this study was provided by the Division of Allied Health Manpower, Department of Health, Education and Welfare.

REFERENCES

1. Meyer, A.: The philosophy of occupational therapy. Arch. Occup. Ther. 1:1, 1922.
2. Slagle, E. C.: Training aides for mental patients. Arch. Occup. Ther. 1:11, 1922.
3. Kielhofner, G. W.: The evolution of knowledge in occupational therapy—understanding adaptation of the chronicaly disabled. Master's Thesis. Department

of Occupational Therapy, University of Southern California, Los Angeles, 1973.
4. Reilly, M.: The modernization of occupational therapy. Am. J. Occup. Ther. 25:243, 1971.
5. Hall, E. T.: The paradox of culture. In Landis, B., and Tauber, E. S. (eds.): In the Name of Life. Holt, Rinehart, and Winston, New York, 1971, p. 226.
6. Henry, J.: Pathways to Madness. Vintage Books (Random House), New York, 1971.
7. White, R.: Strategies of adaptation: an attempt at systematic description. In Coelho, G., et al. (eds.): Coping and Adaptation. Basic Books, New York, 1974.
8. Boulding, K.: The Image, University of Michigan Press, Ann Arbor, 1961.
9. Larrington, G.: An exploratory study of the temporal aspects of adaptive functioning. Master's Thesis. Department of Occupational Therapy, University of Southern California, Los Angeles, California, 1970.
10. DeCharms, R.: Personal Causation. Academic Press, New York, 1968.
11. Dewey, J.: Reconstruction in Philosophy. H. Holt and Company, New York, 1920, p. 36.
12. Hallowell, I.: Culture and Experience. Schocken Books, New York, 1955, p. 217.
13. Hall, E. T.: The Silent Language, Fawcett Publications, Inc., Greenwich, 1959.
14. Parkhurst, H. H.: The cult of chronology. In: Essays in Honor of John Dewey. H. Holt and Company, New York, 1929, p. 23.
15. Toffler, A.: Future Shock. Random House, New York, 1970, p. 360.
16. Reilly, M.: A psychiatric occupational therapy program as a teaching model. Am. J. Occup. Ther. 20:2, 1966.
17. Newcomb, T.: Social Psychology. Henry Holt and Company, New York, 1959.
18. Matsutsuyu, J.: Occupational behavior: a perspective on work and play. Am. J. Occup. Ther. 25:291, 1971.
19. Arensenian, J.: Life cycle factors in mental illness. Ment. Hyg. 52:19, 1968.
20. Kluckhohn, C.: Values and value orientations in the theory of action: an exploration in definition and classification. In Parsons, T., and Shils, E. (eds.): Toward a General Theory of Action. Harvard University Press, Cambridge, 1951.
21. Matsutsuyu, J.: The interest checklist. Am. J. Occup. Ther. 23:323, 1969.
22. Lakein, A.: How to Get Control of Your Time and Your Life. The Signet, The New American Library, Inc., New York, 1974.
23. Kiev, A.: A Strategy of Daily Living. The Free Press, New York, 1973.
24. Black, M. M.: The evolution of social roles—a perspective on fantasy. Master's Thesis. Department of Occupational Therapy, University of Southern California, Los Angeles, California, 1973.

EFFECT OF SENSORY INTEGRATIVE THERAPY ON THE NEUROMOTOR DEVELOPMENT OF RETARDED CHILDREN*

Patricia Montgomery, M.A., and Eileen Richter, B.S.

Three groups of trainable mentally retarded children participated in three different motor programs for an eight-month period. Children receiving sensory integrative therapy showed the greatest gains on test batteries for reflex integration and gross and fine motor skills. Children in a developmental physical education program demonstrated greater improvement on the same test batteries than a third group of children who participated in a recreational, adaptive physical education program and an "arts and crafts" oriented therapy program. Results of data analysis indicate that neuromotor development may be enhanced more effectively by activities which facilitate improved postural responses rather than by practice of specific motor skills.

1.   In the past few years, school systems have become increasingly responsible for the education of mentally retarded children categorized as trainable (below 50 on standard IQ tests). With this new population

---

*Reprinted from *Physical Therapy* (57:799–806, 1977) with permission of the American Physical Therapy Association.

of children has come the need to develop appropriate programs for enhancing motor development.

2.   Traditional approaches to improving motor development such as those described by Kephart[1] and Cratty[2] are geared too high for the trainable mentally retarded child, stress cortical or cognitive learning, are not based on a normal developmental sequence, do not emphasize the importance of sensory functions, and fail to correlate reflex activity and motor skills.

3.   Kinnealey stated that classical academic and behavior modification techniques are based on a level of sensory integration and neurological development which is higher than that present in the mentally retarded child. "Treatment must begin at the sensory stimulation-motor response-sensory feedback level to help facilitate sensorimotor integration."[3]

4.   In a study involving mentally retarded preschool children, the children participating in prescribed sensorimotor activities had statistically significant increments in gross motor, language, and full-scale scores as compared to children participating in randomly selected gross motor tasks.[4] Sensory integration is a specific aspect of sensorimotor functions and "refers to the reception and sorting-out process that is necessary to organize sensory information for use."[5] Sensory integrative therapy, as described by Jean Ayres,[6] can bring about statistically significant increases in academic learning in children with certain types of sensory integrative dysfunction.[7, 8]

5.   Sensorimotor integration refers to the neurologic sequence of sensory input, followed by the integration and sorting-out process which occurs at various levels of the nervous system, a motor response and subsequent sensory input which provides feedback and is again integrated by the nervous system. This cycle of sensory input-motor response-sensory feedback is the substrate of motor skills and higher cognitive abilities.[9] Piaget believes that concrete action precedes and makes possible the use of intellect and that sensorimotor experiences are the foundations of mental development.[10]

6.   Moore has described three types of learning: (1) subcortical (unconscious) learning, (2) reflexive trial-and-error (also unconscious) learning, and (3) cortical (conscious) learning. Learning which occurs unconsciously is easiest and may be most appropriate for therapeutic programs.[9] Remediation aimed at enhancing sensorimotor functions should stress automatic postural responses which do not require the direct attention of the child. Primary emphasis should be placed on appropriate sensory input and therapeutic programs designed to enhance sensory integrative function should precede academic work.[6]

METHOD

7.   Seventy-five children, categorized as trainable mentally retarded (TMR) by the results of intelligence tests, were involved in the study. Fifty children ranging in age from 5 to 12 years comprised the entire population of that age group in one public school and were assigned to one of two experimental groups. Twenty-five TMR children from a private school were matched to the experimental groups by age and served as a control group.

8.   Children with physical handicaps such as cerebral palsy or meningomyelocele were excluded from the study. The school staff identified seven children in the experimental groups and three in the control group who were considered emotionally disturbed or were described as having "autistic tendencies."

9.   Stratified random sampling was used to assign the 50 children at one school to two experimental groups. The children were assigned randomly after being divided by age. For example, of 10 children in one class, the 6-year-olds were assigned randomly to one experimental group (developmental physical education) or the other (sensorimotor program); the remaining 5-year-olds were assigned randomly to the two groups. The 25 children in the control group were matched by age to children in the experimental groups so there would be an equal number of 5-year-olds, 6-year-olds, and so forth in the three groups. Age stratification was necessary for the data analysis because sensory integrative therapy may be more effective for the young child whose brain is more plastic and in the process of forming neural connections.[6] An equal number of children in each classroom was involved in each experimental group to decrease the effect various teachers, teaching procedures, or programs might have on the development of motor skills.

10.   The ratio of boys to girls was 14:11 in the developmental physical education program, 19:6 in the sensorimotor program, and 15:10 in the control group.

11.   Several subjects were dropped from the project because of illness, transfer to another program, or unavailability for evaluation during the scheduled test sessions. Final analyses were completed on 23 subjects in the sensorimotor program, 20 subjects in the developmental physical education program, and 19 subjects in the control group.

12.   The subjects were tested on items which were divided into four categories: (1) gross motor, (2) fine motor, (3) perceptual-motor, and (4) reflex integration. Developmental scales of 60 gross motor items[11] and 35 fine motor items[12] were used. In addition, six items were chosen

from the Frostig Movement Skills Test Battery.[13] A 17-item reflex test, using procedures described by Fiorentino[14] and Ayres,[6] was adapted to a numerical scale.[12]

13.   Testing was completed by four individuals—two occupational therapists, one physical therapist, and one physical education instructor. The physical therapist and one occupational therapist administered the sensorimotor program. The physical education instructor administered the developmental physical education program. The other occupational therapist was not involved in administering either program and was unaware of which children were in each program. The 118 test items were divided among the four testers and each person was responsible for administering the same items during each test session. An attempt to decrease tester bias was made by dividing test items. For example, on the 60-item gross motor battery, the physical education instructor administered 40 items, the physical therapist 10 items, and the occupational therapist 10 items. Scores were recorded on separate forms and compiled when testing was completed. All test sessions were administered in the morning between 9 and 12 o'clock. A pilot study during the previous school year had given each evaluator the opportunity to practice administering specific items. Standard criteria were established for items with poor reliability, and most gross and fine motor items were marked either present or absent, which tended to decrease subjectivity.

14.   Test items themselves were not practiced during the school year by children in either of the experimental groups. Test results were not referred to during the school year and test administrators had little recall as to how children performed on various items.

15.   Although the individuals administering the test had evaluated their own reliability, each child's performance was still subject to variability. Lack of cooperation or understanding complicates test procedures with mentally retarded individuals.

16.   Reflex integration is difficult to assess quantitatively. Responses to test stimuli were considered normal, abnormally present or absent, or somewhere in between. In testing for prone head righting, for example, if the child's head remained flexed when he was suspended in a prone position, the response was marked absent (abnormal). If the head righted to the vertical, the response was marked present (normal). If the head extended, but not to a vertical position, the response was considered "poor." These results were converted to numerical scores to facilitate data analysis—two points for normal integration, one point for "poor" integration, and zero points for an abnormal response.

17.   Test batteries were administered in September 1974 during the first few weeks of the school year. Children in the three groups participated

in their respective programs from September through April. Two test sessions to evaluate progress were administered: one in December 1974 and one in May 1975. An additional test session was completed in the fall of 1975 to measure retention of skill following summer vacation.

PROGRAMS

18.   Children in Experimental Group I were involved in a developmental physical education program three times a week for half-hour sessions.[15] Children in Experimental Group II participated in a therapeutic sensorimotor program three times a week for half-hour sessions.[12] In addition, all children received 16 half-hour swimming lessons during the school year.

19.   The therapy and physical education programs were designed to coordinate with each other by following a normal developmental sequence. Both programs consisted of eight units (approximately four weeks each) of sequenced activities with emphasis on rolling, crawling, creeping, review and variations, sitting balance, kneeling balance, standing balance, and review and variations. Children participated in all activities at the same rate regardless of chronological age or developmental scores.

20.   The therapeutic sensorimotor program placed primary emphasis on sensory input (particularly tactile and vestibular) and activities to enhance reflex integration. The physical education program stressed motor and social aspects of various activities. The difference in programs may be clarified by an example of how rolling activities were used. In the therapeutic program, textured surfaces provided sensory input and rolling up and down inclines was done to facilitate a body righting (on the body) response. In the physical education program, rolling was used in physical fitness activities and in games such as relay races. The ultimate goal of activities in both programs was active movement by the child. Passive patterning was not done.

21.   The control group participated in a physical education program an average of two and one-half times a week for half-hour sessions. This program consisted of randomly selected gross motor activities primarily in a bipedal position. Floor activities were not stressed and a developmental sequence was not followed. The same children also participated in an arts and crafts-oriented occupational therapy program for half-hour sessions an average of two and one-half times a week. Half of the children in the control group received an additional ADL (activities of daily living: dressing) program daily. Swimming was not part of this program.

22.   Class size in all three groups ranged from 6 to 10 children. The staff student ratio in the experimental groups was 1:3 and in the control group 1:4.

RESULTS

23.   Mean scores and standard deviations for the three major test batteries (gross motor, fine motor, and reflex integration) are listed in Table 1. Average changes in scores are computed from fall to winter, winter to spring, and from fall to spring. In all three test batteries, the mean scores of children receiving the therapeutic sensorimotor program improved to a greater extent than scores of children in the other two groups. Children participating in a developmental physical education program improved to a greater extent than children in the control

Table 1

	Total Number of Gross Motor Items Performed								
	Fall		Winter			Spring			
	$\overline{X}$	S.D.	$\overline{X}$	S.D.	$\Delta\overline{X}1$[a]	$\overline{X}$	S.D.	$\Delta\overline{X}2$[b]	$\Delta\overline{X}$[c]
Sensorimotor (Experimental II)	50.6	6.1	51.7	4.0	+1.2	52.4	4.2	+0.7	+1.9
Physical Education (Experimental I)	52.9	3.3	52.8	3.6	−0.1	54.2	3.3	+1.4	+1.3
Control	54.9	4.1	53.3	3.2	−1.6	53.8	2.4	+0.5	−1.1
	Total Number of Fine Motor Items Performed								
	Fall		Winter			Spring			
	$\overline{X}$	S.D.	$\overline{X}$	S.D.	$\Delta\overline{X}1$	$\overline{X}$	S.D.	$\Delta\overline{X}2$	$\Delta\overline{X}$
Sensorimotor (Experimental II)	25.5	4.0	25.7	3.6	+0.2	26.8	4.5	+1.1	+1.3
Physical Education (Experimental I)	26.6	5.4	26.7	3.7	+0.1	26.9	3.9	+0.2	+0.3
Control	28.5	3.3	27.7	2.8	−0.8	28.1	2.7	+0.4	−0.4
	Total Points on Test of Reflex Integration								
	Fall		Winter			Spring			
	$\overline{X}$	S.D.	$\overline{X}$	S.D.	$\Delta\overline{X}1$	$\overline{X}$	S.D.	$\Delta\overline{X}2$	$\Delta\overline{X}$
Sensorimotor (Experimental II)	17.2	4.8	21.5	3.9	+4.3	24.4	3.6	+2.9	+7.2
Physical Education (Experimental I)	19.6	5.8	21.6	4.9	+2.0	22.6	5.1	+1.0	+3.0
Control	19.3	3.4	19.8	3.9	+0.5	20.8	4.6	+1.0	+1.5

[a] $\Delta\overline{X}1$: Mean change—fall to winter.
[b] $\Delta X2$: Mean change—winter to spring.
[c] ΔX: Total mean change—fall to spring.

group. Statistical analyses revealed no significant differences in relation to age or sex.

24.   Bartletts' test[16] for multivariate analysis of variance was done on six variables—differences in total number of gross motor items performed, total number of fine motor items performed, and total score in reflex integration between two test sessions (fall to winter and winter to spring). This is a procedure for testing the null hypothesis with respect to all six variates simultaneously to maintain control over experiment error. Computer Program UMST570 of the University of Minnesota Statistical Program Library was used and computations were done on the University of Minnesota CDC Cyber-74 computer.

25.   The result of the multivariate analysis of variance indicates the null hypothesis (that the mean differences between the three groups were equal) can be rejected. The probability that the differences which occurred were due to chance is less than one in 100 ($p < .01$).

26.   Separate analyses of variance indicated a statistically significant difference among the three groups in the total number of gross motor items performed ($p < .03$) and the total score in reflex integration ($p < .001$). Differences in the number of fine motor items performed were not statistically significant ($p = .27$).

27.   Performance on each test was correlated with performance on subsequent tests and stability coefficients were computed. These figures are listed in Table 2 and indicate that the tests were evaluations of relatively consistent phenomena. These coefficients are, of course, affected by the administration of treatment programs.

28.   Mean scores, standard deviations, and average changes in test scores of the six Frostig perceptual-motor items are shown in Table 3. Stability coefficients are listed in Table 4. Children in the sensorimotor program improved more than children in the other groups in three of six items—block transfer, standing broad jump, and changing body position. Children in the developmental physical education program progressed to a greater extent in bead stringing and sit-ups, and children in the control group progressed more than other children on the number of steps walked on the balance beam.

29.   A factor analysis of items included in the evaluation of reflex integration resulted in three major clusters: (1) equilibrium reactions in prone, supine, and sitting positions; (2) neck righting, asymmetrical and symmetrical tonic neck responses, and tonic labyrinthine responses in prone and supine positions; and (3) lateral and prone head righting responses and protective extension. These clusters of scores generally correlate with the level of central nervous system maturation.[14]

Table 2. Stability coefficients

	Fall to Winter	Winter to Spring	Fall to Spring
GROSS MOTOR ITEMS			
Sensorimotor (Experimental II)	0.78	0.91	0.88
Physical Education (Experimental I)	0.80	0.88	0.83
Control	0.52	0.86	0.49
All Subjects	0.72	0.89	0.77
FINE MOTOR ITEMS			
Sensorimotor (Experimental II)	0.87	0.92	0.90
Physical Education (Experimental I)	0.93	0.85	0.78
Control	0.85	0.68	0.74
All Subjects	0.88	0.84	0.80
REFLEX INTEGRATION			
Sensorimotor (Experimental II)	0.75	0.76	0.63
Physical Education (Experimental I)	0.77	0.86	0.63
Control	0.77	0.56	0.63
All Subjects	0.71	0.75	0.54

DISCUSSION

30.   Test data indicate significant improvement in gross motor skills ($p < .03$) and reflex integration ($p < .001$) in the group of children receiving a therapeutic sensorimotor program. These results, however, should be further verified through additional research. Even though rigid test criteria were used and test examiners made a conscious effort to maintain objectivity, variability in children's performance and observer bias were still possible.

31.   Improvement in reflex integration occurred in all three groups. Comparison of the mean scores in the spring (24.4, 22.6, and 20.8) with a normal score (34), however, indicates that these children were still having pronounced problems with postural responses.

32.   Thirty-five children involved in the study were observed to be tactually defensive during testing. Tactile defensiveness is an integrative deficit in tactile perception which results in aversion to certain types of tactile stimuli. [17] The theory underlying this phenomenon is that the child still retains the original phylogenetic function of tactile stimuli as a warning mechanism. Interpreting tactile stimuli in this manner results in over-alertness or distractibility and "flight-like" behavior. [18]

230

Thirty-three of the 35 children also exhibited an avoiding reaction in the upper extremities (hands).

33. Of 24 children who had inadequate protective extension, 22 exhibited an avoiding reaction, and 14 were considered tactually defensive. Tactile defensiveness may contribute to the persistence of an avoiding reaction which, in turn, interferes with adequate development of protective responses. An avoiding reaction was demonstrated by an additional 13 children who were not considered tactually defensive and who had adequate protective responses.

34. Gains in gross and fine motor skills seem small when viewed as absolutes. It should be remembered that although the children involved in the study were not physically handicapped, they were severely delayed in motor development as determined by comparing their performances on developmental scales with appropriate performances for chronological age. The motor-test items are developmental milestones, so that an improvement on a small number of items indicates a relatively great improvement in the overall functioning of the child.

35. In general, improvements in reflex integration and gross motor skills were greater in the first half of the year. It may be that initial gains were made quickly, followed by slower improvement or that floor activities (using a variety of purposeful tasks in rolling, crawling, and creeping positions) were more effective therapeutic activities than balance activities for this particular sample of children.

36. An indication that children in the sensorimotor group attained a higher level of neuromotor functioning is supported by an analysis of the specific gross and fine motor skills in which the children progressed. These included hopping, alternating feet on stairs, establishment of hand dominance, and use of forefinger pinch—none were practiced and all improved. Stair climbing was never practiced during therapy sessions, yet it is evident that some children reached a higher stage of development by discontinuing "marking time" and using reciprocation when walking up and down stairs. It is hypothesized that the foundation or substrate for this higher level of motor performance was established through improved reflex integration, as indicated by improved scores on reflex testing, and the skill itself developed spontaneously without having to be taught to the child.

37. It is possible to teach a child (cognitively) to alternate feet and walk up and down stairs. He will be able to perform this task as long as his attention is directed to it. When his attention is diverted, however, he may revert to marking time if the foundations for this movement, such as bilateral integration of righting and equilibrium responses, are inadequate to allow him to accomplish the task on an automatic basis.

38. Some motor abilities develop as "splinter skills."[1] Splinter skills are

Table 3. Total change in score on Frostig movement skills test battery (selected items)

ITEM: Number of beads laced within 30 seconds

	Fall $\bar{X}$	Fall S.D.	Winter $\bar{X}$	Winter S.D.	$\Delta\bar{X}1$ [a]	Spring $\bar{X}$	Spring S.D.	$\Delta\bar{X}2$ [b]	$\Delta\bar{X}$ [c]
Sensorimotor (Experimental II)	1.7	1.5	2.0	1.6	+.3	2.5	2.1	+0.5	+0.8
Physical Education (Experimental I)	2.5	1.6	2.9	2.1	+0.4	3.4	2.2	+0.5	+0.9
Control	1.8	1.4	2.1	1.3	+0.3	1.8	1.1	−0.3	0.0

ITEM: Number of blocks transferred within 30 seconds

	Fall $\bar{X}$	Fall S.D.	Winter $\bar{X}$	Winter S.D.	$\Delta\bar{X}1$	Spring $\bar{X}$	Spring S.D.	$\Delta\bar{X}2$	$\Delta\bar{X}$
Sensorimotor (Experimental II)	5.0	2.8	6.1	3.0	+1.1	6.4	3.0	+0.3	+1.4
Physical Education (Experimental I)	6.8	3.5	7.2	3.1	+0.4	7.9	3.3	+0.7	+1.1
Control	6.5	3.2	7.1	2.8	+0.6	6.9	2.8	−0.2	+0.4

ITEM: Distance jumped—standing broad jump (cm)

	Fall $\bar{X}$	Fall S.D.	Winter $\bar{X}$	Winter S.D.	$\Delta\bar{X}1$	Spring $\bar{X}$	Spring S.D.	$\Delta\bar{X}2$	$\Delta\bar{X}$
Sensorimotor (Experimental II)	23.3	22.2	23.5	19.6	+0.2	29.0	24.4	+5.5	+5.7
Physical Education (Experimental I)	27.0	25.9	31.0	28.7	+4.0	29.2	24.0	−1.8	+2.2
Control	36.0	29.2	44.5	26.9	+8.5	35.9	26.0	−8.6	−0.1

ITEM: Number of times child changes body position in 20 seconds

	Fall		Winter		$\Delta\bar{X}1$	Spring		$\Delta\bar{X}2$	$\Delta\bar{X}$
	$\bar{X}$	S.D.	$\bar{X}$	S.D.		$\bar{X}$	S.D.		
Sensorimotor (Experimental II)	1.9	2.1	3.1	2.9	+1.2	3.8	2.9	+0.7	+1.9
Physical Education (Experimental I)	2.7	2.8	3.1	3.0	+0.4	4.5	2.9	+1.4	+1.8
Control	3.7	2.6	4.2	2.5	+0.5	5.3	2.9	+1.1	+1.6

ITEM: Number of sit-ups in 30 seconds

	Fall		Winter		$\Delta\bar{X}1$	Spring		$\Delta\bar{X}2$	$\Delta\bar{X}$
	$\bar{X}$	S.D.	$\bar{X}$	S.D.		$\bar{X}$	S.D.		
Sensorimotor (Experimental II)	0.5	1.6	0.9	2.3	+0.4	0.6	2.0	-0.3	+0.1
Physical Education (Experimental I)	0.9	2.3	0.5	1.6	-0.4	1.1	2.9	+0.6	+0.2
Control	0.5	1.6	1.0	2.6	+0.5	0.5	1.4	-0.5	0.0

ITEM: Number of steps on balance beam

	Fall		Winter		$\Delta\bar{X}1$	Spring		$\Delta\bar{X}2$	$\Delta\bar{X}$
	$\bar{X}$	S.D.	$\bar{X}$	S.D.		$\bar{X}$	S.D.		
Sensorimotor (Experimental II)	2.4	4.4	1.3	2.5	-1.1	1.4	2.5	+0.1	-1.0
Physical Education (Experimental I)	3.2	3.7	2.7	4.1	-0.5	3.1	3.9	+0.4	-0.1
Control	1.3	1.6	1.4	2.7	+0.1	2.1	2.3	+0.7	+0.8

[a] $\Delta\bar{X}1$: Mean change—fall to winter.
[b] $\Delta\bar{X}2$: Mean change—winter to spring.
[c] $\Delta\bar{X}$: Total mean change—fall to spring.

Table 4. Stability coefficients—Frostig test battery

ITEM: Total number of beads strung in 30 seconds	Fall to Winter	Winter to Spring	Fall to Spring
Sensorimotor (Experimental II)	0.86	0.78	0.65
Physical Education	0.88	0.83	0.85
Control	0.70	0.81	0.83
All Subjects	0.83	0.80	0.75
ITEM: Total number of blocks transferred in 30 seconds			
Sensorimotor (Experimental II)	0.73	0.74	0.80
Physical Education	0.88	0.66	0.83
Control	0.79	0.69	0.71
All Subjects	0.81	0.70	0.78
ITEM: Distance of standing broad jump (cm)			
Sensorimotor (Experimental II)	0.68	0.79	0.82
Physical Education (Experimental I)	0.87	0.91	0.92
Control	0.81	0.91	0.82
All Subjects	0.81	0.86	0.85
ITEM: Changing body position— number in 30 seconds			
Sensorimotor (Experimental II)	0.78	0.87	0.63
Physical Education (Experimental I)	0.74	0.85	0.70
Control	0.70	0.78	0.86
All Subjects	0.74	0.84	0.74
ITEM: Number of sit-ups in 30 seconds			
Sensorimotor (Experimental II)	0.62	0.90	0.67
Physical Education (Experimental I)	0.46	0.91	0.30
Control	0.65	0.10	0.35
All Subjects	0.53	0.60	0.41
ITEM: Number of steps on balance beam			
Sensorimotor (Experimental II)	0.70	0.55	0.76
Physical Education (Experimental I)	0.54	0.30	0.49
Control	0.53	0.51	0.54
All Subjects	0.57	0.43	0.57

motor acts learned through repeated practice, and usually require concentration by the child on the individual components of the movement. These skills do not necessarily reflect the child's true motor abilities as they do not generalize to other motor acts and must be practiced to be retained.

39.   Splinter skills may account for the fact that some children lost the ability to do certain tasks from one test session to another. The performance of children in the sensorimotor group deteriorated from fall to spring in the number of steps they could walk on a balance beam (Table 3), possibly because they did not practice this activity. The

balance beam is commonly used for motor training, although it is often too complex for the child's level of development and must be practiced on a cognitive basis.

40.   The performance of other motor skills, such as riding a tricycle or kicking a ball, deteriorated between fall and subsequent test sessions in several children in all three groups. One possible explanation is that children commonly engage in these activities during summer months and, without continued practice during the school year, lose the ability to perform these skills.

41.   Negative changes which occurred over the summer in reflex integration in the sensorimotor group were due primarily to deterioration in equilibrium, head righting, and protective responses. These activities were stressed during the second half of the school year; and because repetition over a period of months is necessary for integration to become firmly established,[6] it is possible that these responses were not well integrated.

42.   On the other hand, children in the developmental physical education program improved over the summer in more reflex items reflecting brain stem responses, those integrated by floor activities stressed in the first half of the year. It may be that these improvements were delayed by-products of improved motor skills or that these children, who were higher functioning as a group, were able to use their enhanced motor abilities more effectively.

43.   Theoretically, the child's adaptive response to sensory input provided by therapeutic procedures will be neural reorganization, a normalizing self-organizing function of the brain.[5, 6] This process probably occurs over a period of months and may continue to enhance function after cessation of treatment. In a study of elementary school children, maintenance of motor skill and continued sensory integration occurred three months following a perceptual-motor program.[19] King stated that motor skills which become automatic (subcortical) should not be subject to regression over periods of time.[20]

44.   The developmental physical education program was designed to produce change through emphasis on motor skills, with reflex integration a by-product of improved skill. The sensorimotor program was designed to improve reflex integration, with motor skill a by-product of more efficient sensorimotor integration. Easton stated that reflexes are the raw materials from which the central nervous system may build volitional movements and hypothesized that muscles engaged in associated movements are functionally connected by reflexes.[21] Data analysis indicates that placing primary emphasis on improving reflex integration is more effective in improving motor skills than placing emphasis on the skills themselves. Traditional motor programs may be

working in reverse in this respect, resulting in slower and less efficient changes in neuromotor development.

CONCLUSIONS

45.   Sensory integrative theory predicts that improvement in sensorimotor integration will result in improvement in motor skills, academic achievements, language abilities, and emotional tone.[6] The results of this study tend to corroborate this theory in regard to motor skills. Language development, academic achievement, and emotional tone were not evaluated, but should be investigated in future studies. The most effective and efficient method of improving motor abilities in children with developmental disabilities appears to be through improvement in primitive postural responses. This may be accomplished best through therapeutic intervention and emphasis on developmental programming. Motor programs which stress motor skills with no regard for the child's level of reflex integration and motor development may result in the acquisition of splinter skills without enhancement of the child's neuromotor development.

ACKNOWLEDGMENT

The authors wish to express appreciation to the following individuals: Molly McEwen, OTR, for assistance in testing; Kris Suhl, Physical Education Instructor, for supervision of one experimental group and assistance in testing; the staff and students at the Child Development Center, St. Paul, Minnesota, and the Louis Whitbeck Fraser School, Inc., Richfield, Minnesota, for their cooperation and participation in the study; and Rod Rosse, Ph.D., Consultant in Research Methods and Data Analysis for Personnel Decisions, Inc., for assistance with the statistical analyses of data.

REFERENCES

1. Kephart, N. C.: The Slow Learner in the Classroom, ed. 2. Charles E. Merrill Publishing Company, Columbus, Ohio, 1971.
2. Cratty, B. J.: Motor Activity and the Education of Retardates. Lea & Febiger, Philadelphia, 1969.
3. Kinnealey, M.: Aversive and non-aversive responses to sensory stimulation in mentally retarded children. Am. J. Occup. Ther. 27:464, 1973.
4. Morrison, D., and Pothier, P.: Two different remedial motor training programs and the development of mentally retarded preschoolers. Am. J. Ment. Defic. 77:251, 1972.
5. Vezie, M. B.: Sensory Integration: A foundation for learning. Academic Therapy Publications (New York) 3:345, 1975.

6. Ayres, A. J.: Sensory Integration and Learning Disorders. Western Psychological Services, Los Angeles, 1972.
7. Ayres, A. J.: Improving academic scores through sensory integration. J. Learning Disabilities 5:336, 1975.
8. Ayres, A. J.: The Effect of Sensory Integrative Therapy on Learning Disabled Children. Published by the Center for the Study of Sensory Integrative Dysfunction, Pasadena, 1976.
9. Moore J.: Concepts from the Neurobehavioral Sciences. Kendall/Hunt Publishing Co., Dubuque, Iowa, 1973.
10. Ginsburg, H., and Opper S · Piaget's Theory of Intellectual Development. Prentice-Hall, Inc., Englewood Cliffs, N.J., 1969.
11. Hoskins, T., and Squires, J.: Development assessment: A test for gross motor and reflex development. Phys. Ther. 53:117, 1973.
12. Montgomery, P., and Richter, E.: Sensorimotor Integration for Developmentally Disabled Children. Western Psychological Services, Los Angeles, 1977.
13. Orpet, R. E.: Frostig Movement Skills Test Battery. Consulting Psychologists Press, Palo Alto, Calif., 1972.
14. Fiorentino, M. R.: Reflex Testing Methods for Evaluating CNS Development, ed 2. Charles C Thomas, Publisher, Springfield, Ill., 1973.
15. Suhl, K.: Developmental Physical Education Curriculum. St. Paul Public Schools, Physical Education Department, St. Paul, Minn., 1974.
16. UMST Statistical Computer Programs Manual. University of Minnesota Computer Center, Minneapolis, 1968.
17. Ayres, A. J.: Patterns of perceptual-motor dysfunction in children: A factor analytic study. Percept. Mot. Skills 20:335, 1965.
18. Ayres, A. J.: Tactile functions: Their relation to hyperactive and perceptual-motor behavior. Am. J. Occup. Ther. 18:6, 1964.
19. McKibbin, E. H.: The effect of additional tactile stimulation in a perceptual-motor treatment program for school children. Am. J. Occup. Ther. 27:191, 1973.
20. King, L. J.: A sensory-integrative approach to schizophrenia. Am. J. Occup. Ther. 28:529, 1974.
21. Easton, T. A.: On the normal use of reflexes. Am. Sci. 60:591, 1972.

DISTRIBUTION OF PERIPHERAL NEUROPATHY IN DIABETIC AMPUTEES*

Otto D. Payton, M.S., and Katherine V. Kemp, M.D.

Motor nerve conduction velocities were recorded on the median, ulnar, radial, peroneal, and tibial nerves of fourteen diabetic, unilateral, lower extremity amputees. The distribution of diabetic neuropathy was investigated and it was concluded that, at a significance level beyond 0.001, the radial nerves were much less likely to be neuropathic than the other nerves studied.

Numerous writers have investigated and reported on the incidence of neuropathy in diabetics using nerve conduction velocity determination as the chief investigative tool. Coers[1] and Ellenberg[2] emphasized the early onset of neuropathy in diabetes. Coers also discussed the histological and morphological findings which accompany the early onset of diabetic neuropathy. The works of numerous investigators have compared the motor nerve conduction velocities of diabetics with that of nondiabetics and have reported a significant lowering of velocity in diabetics. Some differentiated between diabetics with neuropathy and diabetics without neuropathy, and compared them to control subjects. They reported a higher proportion of abnormally low

---

*Reprinted from *Physical Therapy* (51:510–514, 1974) with permission of the American Physical Therapy Association.

values and lower mean values in diabetics, with or without clinical signs of neuropathy, than in apparently healthy persons.[1,3-12]

2.   Gregersen[13] and Gilliatt[14] have established a correlation between sensory loss and reduced motor nerve conduction velocity. Johnson and Waylonis have demonstrated a reduced velocity in the facial nerve of patients with diabetes mellitus.[15] In an interesting study, Eliasson demonstrated a reduction of about 30 percent in the conduction velocity of rats with chemically induced diabetes.[16] He studied both the sensory and motor fibers of the sciatic nerve. This reduction was not corrected with subsequent insulin treatment of the diabetic rats.

3.   None of the literature reviewed included a systematic study of nerve conduction in amputees who were diabetic, none of the studies reviewed included the radial nerve, and the references to any possible pattern of attack of diabetic neuropathy were contradictory or unclear.

PURPOSE

4.   The purpose of this study was to determine whether diabetic neuropathy affects the median, radial, ulnar, peroneal, and tibial nerves equally or differently with regard to motor nerve conduction velocity in diabetic, unilateral, lower extremity amputees. Fagerberg reported 162 conduction velocity measurements on fifty diabetic and thirty-four nondiabetic patients, studying the ulnar and the peroneal nerves.[9] According to his data, if fifty meters per second is the lower limit of normal for the ulnar nerve, 11 percent of his controls fell below this level; 42 percent of the diabetics without clinical neuropathy and 67 percent of the diabetics with clinical neuropathy fell below that level. In the peroneal nerve, if forty meters per second were accepted as the lower limit, 12 percent of the controls fell below this level; 63 percent of the diabetics without neuropathy, and 75 percent of the diabetics with neuropathy fell below this level. He made no further interpretation of these data in terms of differentiation; however, in reporting on his electromyographic studies, he stated that initial signs of motor involvement appeared in the electromyogram of the extensor digitorum brevis muscle, which was the muscle used in recording nerve conduction velocities for the deep peroneal nerve. Gamstorp made 136 measurements on the median, ulnar, and peroneal nerve of twenty-three diabetic children between the ages of three and sixteen years.[17] Of these 136 measurements, one was on a peroneal nerve which was distinctly below normal, one on a median, and seven on peroneal nerves which were low borderline. He concluded that the ulnar velocity was decreased in younger children, and the peroneal velocity was decreased in older children at a significance below the 0.01 level. The

239

differences were highly significant, beyond the 0.001 level, in the peroneal nerve in younger children and the ulnar and median in older children. He stated that these data suggest that the mean values are consistently lower in the legs than in the arms.

5.   Lawrence and Locke reported on motor conduction velocities measured for the ulnar, median, and peroneal nerves of 240 individuals, including 53 controls, 73 diabetics without neuropathy, and 114 diabetics with neuropathy.[18,19] They concluded: "The results indicate that motor nerve fibers are affected in diabetes, that such affection is independent of age and is as great in the upper limb as in the lower."[18] Johnson disputed these results.[20] This disparity of opinion is in need of further investigation.

6.   Eight of the investigations reviewed studied only one or two nerves, and four studied three nerves. Only two reported studies on the median, ulnar, peroneal, and tibial nerves. None included the radial nerve.

METHOD

7.   The subjects were fourteen unilateral lower extremity amputees who were diabetic. All patients fitting this description who were active cases in the outpatient physical therapy clinic of the University of Maryland Hospital during the time of the study were included except for one patient who was overlooked. Some patients were selected at the time of their return to the prosthetic clinic for routine follow-up.

8.   Motor nerve conduction velocities were recorded for the median, ulnar, and radial nerves bilaterally and for the peroneal and tibial nerves on the nonamputated, lower extremity for each subject, a total of 112 measurements. For uniformity, the techniques described by Honet and Jebsen were used exclusively.[21] A general purpose, twenty-three-gauge, tapered, coaxial needle electrode was used. In each case, proper needle placement was checked by electromyography before the conduction study proceeded. For the median nerve, the needle was placed in the abductor pollicis brevis muscle. The proximal stimulus point was just proximal to the elbow and medial to the bicipital tendon, and the distal stimulus point was at the wrist between the palmaris longus and the flexor carpi radialis tendons. For the ulnar nerve, the needle was placed in the abductor digiti minimi. The proximal stimulus point was the ulnar groove on the medial aspect of the elbow, and the distal stimulus point was volar and proximal to the ulnar styloid. For the radial nerve, the needle was placed in the extensor indicis which was located four centimeters proximal and one centimeter lateral to the ulnar styloid. The proximal stimulus point was the groove between the brachialis and brachioradialis, and the distal

240

stimulus point was six or seven centimeters proximal and one to two centimeters lateral to the ulnar styloid. For the peroneal nerve, the needle was placed in the extensor digitorum brevis in the dorsal, proximal, lateral quadrant of the foot. The proximal stimulus point was behind the fibular neck and the distal point was just lateral to the tibialis anterior tendon. For the tibial nerve, the needle was placed in the abductor hallucis. The proximal stimulus point was the medial popliteal fossa, and the distal stimulus point was posterior to the medial malleolus.

9.   An electromyograph was used which had an automatic conduction time indicator attached.* Distal time in milliseconds was subtracted from proximal time, and this difference was divided into the distance between the two stimulus points recorded in millimeters. The result was the conduction velocity in meters per second.

10.   Prior to the beginning of the experiment, the standards of Honet and Jebsen were accepted as definitions of normal range for motor velocity.[21] They reported the following normal ranges: median nerve, forty-five to seventy-five meters per second; ulnar, forty-five to seventy-five meters per second; radial, forty-five to eighty meters per second; peroneal, thirty-eight to sixty-five meters per second; tibial, thirty-eight to sixty-five meters per second. For the purpose of this study, any obtained velocity which measured higher than the lower limits reported by Honet and Jebsen was considered not to be indicative of a neuropathy. These lower limits are well below the averages reported by seven writers summarized by Lawrence and Locke[19]; therefore, according to the literature, velocities recorded below these lower limits should be clearly neuropathic.

11.   Since the principal hypothesis to be tested was that the distribution of neuropathy for the eight nerves would not be different from an equal proportional distribution, the principal statistical tool was chi-square for a single sample, goodness-of-fit design.[22]

RESULTS

12.   The age range for the group of fourteen subjects was forty-eight to eighty-three years with a mean age of 63.2. The mean length of time since onset of diabetes was 12.3 years with a range of one to thirty years. In all cases, the diabetes was well under control at the time of testing. The diabetes was controlled with chlorpropamide (Diabenese®) for three patients, insulin for six patients, tolbutamide (Orinase®) for two patients, diet alone for two patients, and phenformin HCL (DBI®)

---

*Teca", Model TE 2-7.

for one patient. The results were recorded for the indicated nerve on the amputated side or on the nonamputated side, rather than left or right.

13.   Table 1 shows the observed distribution of neuropathy in sixty observations of the eight nerves studied, and the computation of the total chi-square adjusted for subject variability. The resulting statistic was 37.74 with 7 degrees of freedom, which is significant beyond the 0.001 level, that is, there is less than one chance in a thousand that the observed frequencies could occur by chance. The neuropathy was not proportionately distributed among the eight nerves studied.

14.   From an inspection of the raw data alone, the radial nerves could logically have made the largest contribution to the total chi-square. To confirm this assumption and to clarify the exact location of the disproportionality demonstrated by the principal test, the over-all chi-square was decomposed into its component parts and adjusted for subject variability. This was accomplished by means of an orthogonal contrast matrix.[23] In this manner, each contribution to the total chi-square could be delineated and contrasted to demonstrate clearly the sources of the inequality. Table 2 illustrates these components of the chi-square attributable to contrasts, and adjusted for subject variability. The contrast between the radial nerves and the other six nerves is

Table 1. Chi-square analysis: overall comparison of eight nerves in fourteen unilateral, lower extremity amputees with diabetes

Nerve	Observed	Expected	$O = E$[a]	$(O = E)^2$[b]
Amputated side				
Median	10	7.5	2.5	6.25
Ulnar	10	7.5	2.5	6.25
Radial	1	7.5	−6.5	42.25
Nonamputated				
Median	10	7.5	2.5	6.25
Ulnar	5	7.5	−2.5	6.25
Radial	2	7.5	−5.5	30.25
Peroneal	10	7.5	2.5	6.25
Tibial	12	7.5	4.5	20.25
TOTAL	60	60.0	. . .	124.00

[a]"Observed" minus "expected."
[b]χ^2 adjusted for subject variability:

$$\frac{124.00}{\left(\frac{60 - 296/7}{8}\right)} = \frac{124.00}{3.28} = 37.74$$

Table 2. Components of χ^2 attributable to contrasts (adjusted for subject variability) in comparison of eight nerves in fourteen unilateral lower extremity diabetic amputees

Contrast		df	p
Radial nerves vs. others	29.23	1	0.001
Median nerves	0.00	1	NS
Ulnar nerves	3.80	1	0.10
Radial nerves	0.15	1	NS
Peroneal vs. tibial	0.61	1	NS
2 ulnar vs. 2 radial nerves	1.90	1	NS
Median and ulnar nerves vs. peroneal and tibial	2.05	1	NS
Between All Sites	37.74	7	0.001

significant beyond the 0.001 level. No other contrasts were statistically significant, although the contrast between the two ulnar nerves is of some interest. The observed difference in the distribution of neuropathy over the two ulnar nerves could occur by chance in one sample out of ten, which is not generally believed to be a significant difference. No other contrasts were significant.

DISCUSSION

15.   On the basis of the evidence presented here, one could logically conclude that the diabetic amputee is much less likely to demonstrate a neuropathy in the radial nerves than in the median, ulnar, peroneal, or tibial nerves. The reason for this disproportionality was not investigated here, but it would be an interesting topic for investigation. Although the discrepancy between the two ulnar nerves is not significant according to the usual standards for statistical significance, the differences are still large enough to cause the writers to speculate about a possible tendency for neuropathy to proceed to the arm on the amputated side before attacking the arm on the nonamputated side. Such a tendency was not established by this study, but the present study does raise the question for further investigation. The evidence may be obscured by the wide range in time since onset of diabetes in the cases reported here. If the length of time since onset for all the patients had been more comparable, a clearer pattern of attack might have been evident. This would seem to be a topic worthy of further investigation.

16.   Unilateral amputees, ideally, should be completely independent on

crutches before prosthetic prescription or before gait training on a pylon. Most of the upper extremity antigravity muscles which are used in crutch ambulation are supplied by the radial nerves. The present study suggests that the radial nerve is much less frequently attacked by diabetic neuropathy or is attacked last among the nerves here studied. One may, therefore, logically conclude that even amputees with generalized diabetic neuropathy will probably be able to ambulate safely with crutches. This point has been supported by the clinical experience of the authors.

SUMMARY

17. The distribution of peripheral neuropathy was investigated in a sample of fourteen unilateral lower extremity amputees with diabetes. Motor nerve conduction velocities were determined for the median, radial, and ulnar nerves bilaterally, and the peroneal and tibial nerves on the remaining lower extremity. At a significance level beyond 0.001, the radial nerves were found to be less likely to be neuropathic than the other nerves studied. Possibilities for further research were indicated, as well as the clinical significance of the present report.

ACKNOWLEDGMENT

J. Richard Hebel, Ph.D., did the statistical analysis reported in this study.

REFERENCES

1. Coers, C., and Hildebrand, J.: Latent neuropathy in diabetes and alcoholism. Neurology 15:19, 1965.
2. Ellenberg, M.: Diabetic neuropathy presenting as the initial clinical manifestation of diabetes. Ann. Intern. Med. 49:620, 1958.
3. Chopra, J. S., and Hurwitz, I. J.: Femoral nerve conduction in diabetes and chronic occlusive vascular disease. J. Neurol. Neurosurg. Psychiat. 31:28, 1968.
4. Wakamatsu, H., and Wako, A.: Motor nerve conduction velocity in diabetes mellitus, relation with arteriosclerosis, blood sugar, arterial blood PH, serum electrolytes and tissue temperature. Electromyography 7:185, 1967.
5. Gregersen, G.: Diabetic neuropathy: Influence of age, sex, metabolic control, and duration of diabetes on motor conduction velocity. Neurology 17:972, 1967.
6. Skillman, T. G., et al.: Motor nerve conduction velocity in diabetes mellitus. Diabetes 10:46, 1961.
7. Ferrari-Forcade, A., et al.: Estudio della velocidad de conduccion nerviosa en la diabetes. Acta Neurol. Lat. Am. 6:43, 1960.
8. Gregersen, G.: Latency time, maximal amplitude and electromyography in diabetic patients. Acta Med. Scand. 183:55, 1968.
9. Fagerberg, S. E., et al.: Motor disturbances in diabetes mellitus. Acta Med. Scand. 174:711, 1963.
10. Locke, S., et al.: Diabetic amyotrophy. Am. J. Med. 34:775, 1963.

11. Mayer, R. F.: Nerve conduction studies in man. Neurology 13:1021, 1963.
12. Mulder, D. W., et al.: The neuropathies associated with diabetes mellitus. Neurology 11:275, 1961.
13. Gregersen, G.: Vibratory perception threshold and motor conduction velocity in diabetics and non-diabetics. Acta Med. Scand. 183:61, 1968.
14. Gilliatt, R. W., and Willison, R. G.: Peripheral nerve conduction in diabetic neuropathy. J. Neurol. Neurosurg. Psychiat. 25:11, 1962.
15. Johnson, E. W., and Waylonis, G. W.: Facial nerve conduction delay in patients with diabetes mellitus. Excerpta Medicus 2203, 1965.
16. Eliasson, G. S.: Nerve conduction changes in experimental diabetes. J. Clin. Invest. 43:2353, 1964.
17. Gamstorp, I.: Conduction velocity of peripheral motor nerves in mental retardation, diabetes and various neurological diseases in childhood. Acta Pediat. Scand. 53:408, 1964.
18. Lawrence, D. G., and Locke, S.: Motor nerve conduction velocity in diabetes. Arch. Neurol. 5:483, 1961.
19. Lawrence, D. G., and Locke, S.: Letter. Arch. Neurol. 7:365, 1962.
20. Johnson, E. W.: Motor nerve conduction velocity in diabetes. Arch. Neurol. 7:385, 1962.
21. Honet, J. C., and Jebsen, R. H.: Electrodiagnosis, Part II: What peripheral nerve stimulation shows. Resident Physician 15:105, 1969.
22. Siegel, S.: Non-Parametric Statistics for the Behavioral Sciences. McGraw-Hill Book Company, New York, 1956.
23. Sokal, R. R., and Rohlf, F. J.: Biometry: The Principles and Practice of Statistics in Biological Research. W. H. Freeman, San Francisco, 1969.

COMPARISON OF THE HOLD-RELAX PROCEDURE AND PASSIVE MOBILIZATION ON INCREASING MUSCLE LENGTH*

Marvin C. Tanigawa, M.A.

Thirty normal male subjects were used in this study to compare the effects of the proprioceptive neuromuscular facilitation (PNF) hold-relax procedure and passive mobilization on tight hamstring muscles. A mathematical method was used to measure the angle of passive straight leg raising rather than the goniometric method. The study demonstrated that subjects receiving the PNF hold-relax procedure increased their range of passive straight leg raising to a higher degree and at a faster rate than the subjects receiving passive mobilization.

1.   The prevention of deformity and the preservation of function are of major concern to the physical therapist, and, to meet these goals, much time is spent improving or maintaining a patient's joint range of motion. Many methods of lengthening shortened soft tissue are available; the question centers on which method produces the greatest increase in the range of motion of joints with imitation. The purpose of

---

*Reprinted from *Physical Therapy* (52:725–734, 1972) with permission of the American Physical Therapy Association. Photographs have been omitted.

this study is to compare two mobilization techniques which are currently in use: passive mobilization and the PNF hold-relax procedure.

2. In passive mobilization, the stretching force is applied independently of any active movement by the patient.[1] The stretching force may be applied by devices such as braces and splints or manually by the therapist.

3. PNF may be defined as a method "of promoting or hastening the response of the neuromuscular mechanism through stimulation of the proprioceptors."[2] Hold-relax is one of the PNF techniques used to increase joint range of motion and is based upon an isometric contraction of the shortened muscle performed against maximal resistance. No joint movement should occur, and the isometric contraction must not be overcome. The hold-relax procedure is performed at any point in the subject's range of motion where limitation is present as a result of pain, muscle spasm, or other causes. At the point of limitation, the muscle is placed on a slight degree of tension so the muscle will be able to perform a maximal isometric contraction as indicated by the length-tension principle.[3]

METHOD

Subjects

4. Thirty normal male subjects between 20 and 48 years of age were selected and were divided equally by random distribution into a control group, a passive mobilization group, and a PNF hold-relax group. The mean age of the subjects in the control group was 27.4 years; in the passive mobilization group, 23.5 years; and in the PNF hold-relax group, 25.7 years.

5. The basic criterion for subject selection was passive straight leg raising of less than 70 degrees in the right lower limb. The angle of passive straight leg raising was observed with the subject supine with the right lower limb elevated passively until the subject stated that he felt a pull in the popliteal fossa of that limb. The perception of this pull was used as the indicator that the angle of maximum passive straight leg raising had been reached and that the hamstring muscles were taut. All measurements and treatments were performed on the subject's right lower limb.

Measurements

6. To accurately measure the angle of passive straight leg raising, a mathematical method involving the calculation of the sine of a right

angle triangle was used rather than the goniometric method. For this calculation, the following measurements were necessary: (1) leg length measured from the greater trochanter to the lateral malleolus, (2) the distance from the greater trochanter to the floor, and (3) the distance from the lateral malleolus to the floor.

7. A plumb line was constructed using an eight ounce (0.24 kg) plumb and a tape measure calibrated to an eighth of an inch (0.42 cm). The plumb line was suspended by the examiner so that it remained taut while the tip of the plumb just touched the floor. All measurements were read to the nearest eighth of an inch (0.42 cm).

8. Two bony landmarks were identified with the subject supine. The greater trochanter and the lateral malleolus of the right lower limb were palpated, and the greatest prominence of these landmarks was marked with an indelible felt tip marker.

9. Two measurements were taken with the subject supine. A measurement of leg length was taken by measuring the distance from the mark on the greater trochanter to the mark on the lateral malleolus. Secondly, a measurement from the great trochanter to the floor was taken at that point where the mark on the greater trochanter intersected the taut plumb line.

10. While determining the distance from the lateral malleolus to the floor, the left knee was flexed over the edge of the table and was maintained at a 90-degree angle by placing a strap around the table legs. This was done to prevent excessive lumbar spine movement and posterior pelvic rotation which could influence the angle of straight leg raising.

11. Prior to elevating the right limb, the examiner instructed the subject to relax his entire limb and to allow the examiner to passively elevate the limb. The subject was also instructed to verbally inform the examiner the moment he perceived a pull in the popliteal fossa.

12. The examiner passively elevated the subject's right limb with his left hand around the posterior aspect of the subject's ankle proximal to the lateral malleolus. While elevating the limb with his left hand at a slow rate, the examiner held a taut plumb line with his right hand next to the mark on the lateral malleolus. At the moment the subject expressed the perception of a pull in the popliteal fossa, the examiner observed the point at which the mark on the lateral malleolus intersected the plumb line.

Calculation of the Angle of Passive Straight Leg Raising

13. As the sine of an angle in a right angle triangle is equal to the ratio of the length of the side opposite the angle to the length of the hypot-

enuse, the formula to calculate the angle of passive straight leg raising is as follows: the sine of the angle θ is equivalent to the ratio of the perpendicular distance from the lateral malleolus to the level of the greater trochanter (the difference of the distance from the lateral malleolus to the floor and from the greater trochanter to the floor) to the length of the leg (the distance from the greater trochanter to the lateral malleolus). The angle θ can then be determined from a table of natural trigonometric functions.

Procedures

14.   All subjects were seen two days per week on a Monday-Thursday or a Tuesday-Friday schedule for four consecutive weeks. The subjects in the two treatment groups were measured prior to and after treatment on day 1 through day 6; the control subjects were also measured twice on day 1 through day 6. On day 7, all subjects were seen only to check the markings on the greater trochanter and the lateral malleolus; these marks were darkened as had been done on the previous testing days. On day 8, all subjects were placed in the positions for measurement, and one measurement of passive straight leg raising was obtained.
15.   All subjects were told to refrain from intentional stretching of their hamstring muscles, but to continue with normal activities. A metronome calibrated to one beat per second was used as a timing apparatus for all procedures.

PNF Hold-Relax Procedure

16.   For this study, two lower limb PNF patterns were used. For each procedure, the subject's limb was taken passively by the examiner in a direction opposite to the resistance being applied.
17.   Knott and Voss describe pattern 1 as follows: With the subject's knee extended, the examiner resists hip extension, abduction, and internal rotation, plantar flexion with eversion, and toe flexion.[2] To resist pattern 1, the palmar surface of the examiner's right hand and fingers exert pressure on the lateral aspect of the plantar surface of the subject's foot and toes. The palmar surface of the examiner's left hand and fingers exert pressure on the posterolateral aspect of the subject's thigh proximal to the popliteal fossa.
18.   With the subject supine, pattern 1 was demonstrated once passively on the right limb to indicate the direction of movement desired. The following instructions were given to the subject: "Just relax your leg, and let me raise it. I want you to let me know when you first notice a pull behind your knee. When I say 'Push!' I want you to try to push

249

your leg down towards me as hard as you can, pushing your foot against my hand at the same time. I'll be pushing against your leg and foot to keep you from moving. You can hold the table to stabilize yourself." Using the manual contacts for pattern 1, the examiner passively elevated the subject's limb into hip flexion, adduction, and external rotation, dorsiflexion with inversion, and toe extension; the knee was kept in extension. Further passive elevation was stopped when the subject stated that he felt a pull in the popliteal fossa. The command, "Push!" was given, and pattern 1 was held isometrically for seven seconds, followed by five seconds of rest during which the limb was lowered to the table. The procedure for pattern 1 was repeated a second time followed by a period of rest.

19. Pattern 2 is described by Knott and Voss as follows: With the subject's knee extended, the examiner resists hip extension, adduction, and external rotation, plantar flexion with inversion, and toe flexion.[2] To resist the pattern, the examiner's left hand and fingers exert pressure on the medial aspect of the plantar surface of the subject's foot and toes. The palmar surface of the examiner's right hand and fingers exert pressure on the posteromedial aspect of the subject's thigh proximal to the popliteal fossa.

20. The instructions to the subject and the procedure for pattern 2 were identical to pattern 1 except that the subject's right limb was passively elevated into hip flexion, abduction, and internal rotation, foot and ankle dorsiflexion with eversion, and toe extension. The subject was instructed to pull his right leg down toward his left leg when the command, "Pull!" was given, and pattern 2 was resisted.

Passive Mobilization Procedure

21. The subject was supine with a strap, 5.1 centimeters wide, placed over the left thigh 5.1 centimeters proximal to the patella, under the right thigh, and fastened securely to the table. The strap was used to stabilize the pelvis as the contralateral limb was being mobilized.

22. Facing the subject, the examiner placed the subject's right limb on his right shoulder and cupped his hands over the medial and lateral aspects of the subject's knee to maintain full knee extension. The following instructions were given: "Just relax your leg and foot, and let me raise your leg. Let me know as soon as you feel a pull behind your knee. At this point, I'm going to push your leg up for two seconds and hold it there for five seconds. I'll then lower your leg for five seconds and repeat the procedure three times more."

23. The subject's limb was elevated until a pull was felt in the popliteal

fossa. The limb was further elevated at a moderate rate for two seconds and held in that position for five seconds. The limb was then lowered for five seconds of rest. The procedure was repeated three more times.

Control Procedure

24.   The control subjects were placed in the positions for measurement, and a measurement for passive straight leg raising was obtained. The subjects were allowed to rest on the table with both knees flexed over the edge of the table for forty-five seconds, after which time a second set of measurements was obtained.

ANALYSIS OF DATA

The Immediate Effects Observed

25.   To determine the immediate effects observed, the mean of the difference between the two measurements taken on the subjects on each treatment day was calculated. The subjects in the PNF hold-relax group consistently had the greatest gain in the range of passive straight leg raising on each treatment day; the passive mobilization group had consistently greater daily gains than the control group. The mean daily gain for the PNF hold-relax group was 7.6 degrees; for the passive mobilization group, 4.5 degrees; and for the control group, 0.7 degrees. Figure 1 depicts the immediate mean gain in the range of passive straight leg raising made by each group on each treatment day. Each point on the figure represents the mean gain made by a particular group on a particular day of treatment.

Cumulative Effects From Day 1 to Day 6

26.   The cumulative effects of six days of mobilization are presented in Table 1, which indicates the mean range of passive straight leg raising for each group when initially measured on day 1 and when finally measured after mobilization on day 6. The PNF hold-relax group showed the greatest increase in range of the three groups. The increase attained by the PNF hold-relax group was 2.2 times greater than that of the passive mobilization group, and 11.3 times greater than that of the control group. The passive mobilization group increased its range 5.1 times more than the control group.

251

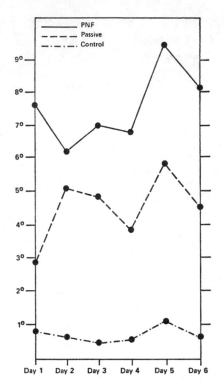

Figure 1. The immediate daily mean gains in the range of passive straight leg raising (Fig. 7 in original article)

Effects of Seven Days Without Mobilization

27.   Table 2 presents data on the effects on the range of passive straight leg raising from day 6 to day 8—one week without mobilization. The measurement on day 6 is the measurement taken after mobilization, and the day 8 measurement is the single measurement taken after

Table 1. Cumulative effects of treatment for day 1 through day 6

Group N = 10 per group	Mean Degrees of Passive SLR on Day 1	Mean Degrees of Passive SLR on Day 6	Mean Degrees of Gain or Loss from Day 1 to Day 6
PNF hold-relax	35.2	51.1	+15.9
Passive mobilization	32.1	39.2	+7.1
Control	35.6	37.0	+1.4

SLR = straight leg raising.

Table 2. The effects of seven days without mobilization

Group N = 10 per group	Mean Degrees of Passive SLR on Day 6	Mean Degrees of Passive SLR on Day 8	Mean Degrees of Gain or Loss from Day 6 to Day 8
PNF hold-relax	51.1	44.9	−6.2
Passive mobilization	39.2	33.9	−5.3
Control	37.0	35.7	−1.3

SLR = straight leg raising.

seven days without mobilization. All groups showed a decrease in the range of passive straight leg raising as a result of seven days without mobilization. Although the PNF hold-relax group had the greatest loss, the loss of that group was just 0.9 degree more than the passive mobilization group.

Cumulative Effects From Day 1 to Day 8

28.   The cumulative effects of mobilization from day 1 to day 8 represent six days of mobilization followed by one week without mobilization (Table 3). The measurement for day 1 is the initial measurement taken before mobilization is initiated, and the day 8 measurement is the final one taken after one week without mobilization. All groups showed an increase in the range of passive straight leg raising with the PNF hold-relax group showing the greatest gain. The gain attained by the PNF hold-relax group was 5.4 times greater than the passive mobilization group and 97 times greater than the control group; the passive mobilization group's gain was 18 times more than the control group.

29.   Figure 2 shows the cumulative effects of mobilization on the range of passive straight leg raising observed in the three groups for the entire testing period of four weeks. The points in the figure represent the

Table 3. Cumulative effects of mobilization for the entire test period

Group N = 10 per group	Mean Degrees of Passive SLR on Day 1	Mean Degrees of Passive SLR on Day 8	Mean Degrees of Gain or Loss from Day 1 to Day 8
PNF hold-relax	35.2	44.9	+9.7
Passive mobilization	32.1	33.9	+1.8
Control	35.6	35.7	+0.1

SLR = straight leg raising.

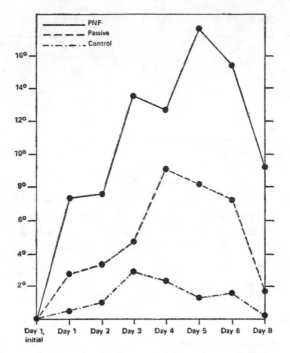

Figure 2. The cumulative gains in the range of passive straight leg raising (Fig. 8 in original article)

mean values of the range taken initially on day 1 and the mean values obtained each day after mobilization, and, in the case of the control group, they represent the mean of the second measurement taken each day. The mean of the initial measurement taken on day 1 for each group is considered as the base and is subtracted from itself and from the means of the respective groups on the various treatment days so all groups would start at zero degrees of passive straight leg raising.

Analysis of Variance

30.   To test the null hypothesis that the two mobilization procedures had no significant effect on increasing the muscle length of tight hamstring muscles as compared to the control subjects, the following variables were considered in an analysis of variance: the effects of the treatment, the influence of the treatment days, the interaction between treatment and treatment days, the contrast between the two treatments, and the contrast between subjects receiving mobilization and the control subjects. Table 4 presents the variables considered and their variance ratios (F values).

254

Table 4. F values as determined by analysis of variance

Variables	F-values	F-value needed for 5 percent significance	F-value needed for 0.1 percent significance
Treatment	27.63[a]		6.91
Days	2.12	2.27	
Interaction	0.55	1.88	
PNF hold-relax vs. passive mobilization	21.15[a]		10.83
Mobilization vs. control	34.10[a]		10.83

[a]Significant at the 0.1 percent level of significance.

31. At a 0.1 percent level of significance, the F values reveal that the three treatment groups were not equal in their ability to effect a change in their range of passive straight leg raising as a result of being subjects in this study. The influence of the days was not significant even at the 5 percent level, which meant that the effect of the days was not significant in this study. The interaction effect was not significant, suggesting that the treatment effect and the day effect functioned independently of each other. At a level of significance greater than 0.1 percent, the analysis indicated that all subjects receiving mobilization increased their range of passive straight leg raising more than the control subjects. Finally, the analysis showed that, at a level of significance greater than 0.1 percent, the PNF hold-relax procedure was a more effective method for increasing the length of tight hamstring muscles than the passive mobilization procedure over the entire test period.

Days Necessary to Effect a Significant Increase in Range

32. To determine the number of days necessary to effect a statistically significant increase in the range of passive straight leg raising, a standard one-tailed t test was perfomed between the mean range of passive straight leg raising of the treatment groups and the control group on the days of treatment. The calculated t value had to exceed 1.73 (the t value at 5 percent significance) or 2.54 (the t value at 1 percent significance) in order to be considered significant at the respective levels.

33. Table 5 presents the calculated t values between the PNF hold-relax group and the control group and between the passive mobilization group and the control group on the days of treatment. Day 1 is excluded because the data are artificial. The passive mobilization group

255

Table 5. t values as determined by t tests between the treatment groups and the control group on each treatment day

Group	Day 2	Day 3	Day 4	Day 5	Day 6
1[a]	2.41[c]	2.98[d]	2.38[c]	3.42[d]	3.31[d]
2[b]	0.84	0.62	1.18	1.69	1.88[c]

[a]Group 1—PNF hold-relax group vs. control group.
[b]Group 2—passive mobilization group vs. control group.
[c]Significant at the 5 percent level of significance.
[d]Significant at the 1 percent level of significance.

never reached the 1 percent level of significance, whereas the PNF hold-relax group reached the 1 percent level on day 3 and remained at that level after day 5.

Linear Regression

34.　A linear regression, which examines the correlation between two variables, was performed to test the correlation between the treatment period and the cumulative effect of mobilization on the two treatment groups. This was done because the effect of the day variable in the analysis of variance was barely insignificant at the 5 percent level.

Figure 3 plots the mean range of passive straight leg raising after mobilization for the two treatment groups, and the least squares line for each group.

35.　A correlation existed between the cumulative range of passive straight leg raising and the treatment days at the 1 percent level of significance, which meant that the cumulative effect of mobilization was dependent on the number of days of mobilization. A t test performed between the two slopes of the least squares line derived from the linear regression was significant at the 1 percent level of significance, which meant that the cumulative range of the PNF hold-relax group increased at a faster rate than that of the passive mobilization group.

DISCUSSION

36.　The large gains in range achieved by the PNF hold-relax group might be explained by autogenic inhibition and active mobilization of connective tissue. Kabat states that relaxation of shortened muscles can be brought about by a maximal isometric contraction of that muscle in a position of slight stretch as is done in the PNF hold-relax pro-

256

\

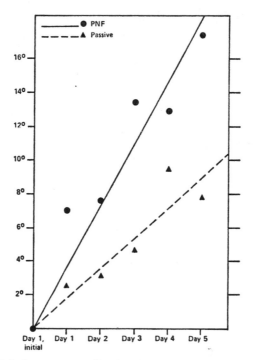

Figure 3. Plot of the least squares line for the PNF hold-relax group and the passive mobilization group (Fig. 9 in original article)

cedure.[4] Although Kabat does not explain the neurophysiological mechanism involved in this phenomenon, autogenic inhibition may be a possible explanation.

37.   Autogenic inhibition, as defined by Ruch and Patton, is "...inhibition mediated by afferent fibers from a stretched muscle and acting on the motoneurons supplying the stretched muscle..."; in other words, the muscle being stretched is inhibited and is caused to relax.[5] It is hypothesized that the Golgi tendon organs (GTOs) are involved in this inhibition.

38.   When an extreme stretch is applied to a muscle, the GTOs are believed to become stimulated and to transmit impulses to an interneuron in the spinal cord which inhibits the alpha motor neuron of the muscle being stretched. These impulses override the impulses from the muscle spindle and cause the muscle to relax suddenly.[6] Houk and Hennemann found, contrary to belief, that the GTOs are very sensitive to active contractions of muscle.[7] The GTOs thus respond to both shortening and extension of muscle.[8] During a maximal isometric contraction with the muscles in their lengthened range, therefore, a great

257

amount of tension is produced which may stimulate the GTOs in the hamstring muscles, causing them to reflexly relax; however, no physiological information is available as to how long this inhibition persists.

39. An active stretch of the connective tissues joining the muscles to their attachments as they perform a maximal isometric contraction may also explain the gains seen in the PNF hold-relax group. During an isometric contraction, the development of maximal tension is related to the development of maximal interaction between the contractile elements of muscle tissue.[8] Because of the interaction of the contractile elements, the tension produced during an isometric contraction will probably be exerted on the connective tissue involved with the muscle, pulling primarily on the connective tissue attachments of the hamstring muscles. Stretching of these attachments could possibly explain the long-term effects described in this study.

40. Although not high, the gain in the range of the passive mobilization group was satisfactory. The gain may be a result of a mechanical stretch of the shortened structures. Soft tissues, such as muscle, ligaments, tendons, and fascia are extensible to a certain degree. Passive mobilization relies on the extensibility of these tissues in order to increase the range of motion of limited joints.

41. The GTO reflex may also be one of the factors responsible for the gains seen in the passive mobilization group. One might conjecture that passive mobilization could activate the GTO reflex and cause partial inhibition of the hamstring muscles, allowing an increase in the range of motion. Neurophysiology studies have shown that the GTO reflex can be activated by a great amount of passive stretch, though not to the high level seen in a maximally resisted isometric contraction.

42. There is a question of the myotatic reflex being triggered when the hamstring muscles are mobilized. It seems logical that passive mobilization could activate the muscle spindle and cause the hamstring muscles to reflexly contract and prevent any gain in the range of straight leg raising past the point of limitation.[6] Levine and coworkers found, however, that passive stretching increased the range of motion of patients with spasticity.[9]

43. A phenomenon reported by a number of subjects in the passive mobilization group was the production of gain when passive mobilization was applied to tight hamstring muscles. A pain stimulus can produce a reflex spasm of the local muscle and cause it to shorten.[6] Such a response may have prevented further gains in the passive mobilization group. According to Adams, "the pain associated with passive [mobili-

zation] of [shortened muscles] suggests that the change is primarily in the elastic supporting tissues," resulting in damage to the sarcolemma.[10] Such damage may result in fibrous changes, further limiting the extensibility of the muscle.

44.   The improvement in the control group could be a result of the physical act of passively elevating the subject's limb until the perception of a pull in the popliteal fossa was felt; each time the limb was elevated, a slight amount of passive mobilization might have been involved. The improvement in range could also have been the result of the halo effect reported in psychology literature; the fact that the subject was involved in a study to determine the increases in the range of motion was enough incentive to cause the observed increases in the control group.

45.   The loss in the range of motion seen in the three groups was probably the result of discontinuing straight leg raising at the end of the subject's range. To maintain mobility throughout full range, the joints involved have to be exercised regularly through the full range of motion.

46.   With vigorous stretching, the sarcolemma and other connective tissues associated with muscles may have been damaged, particularly in the passive mobilization group where pain upon mobilization was reported. This damage might have led to fibrous changes during the week without mobilization resulting in a decrease in the extensibility of the muscles and a loss in the range of passive straight leg raising.

CONCLUSION

47.   On the basis of the findings within the limits of this study, one can conclude that the PNF hold-relax procedure is a much more effective method for increasing the range of motion of shortened tissue than passive mobilization. The PNF hold-relax procedure results in greater increases in range and at a faster rate than the passive mobilization procedure.

48.   The choice of method with a patient will depend upon the physical therapist's discretion. The PNF hold-relax procedure is preferred because the patient is actively participating in his treatment which is psychologically healthier for him and because the likelihood of damage to the muscle and its supporting connective tissue is less. Because this method utilizes an isometric contraction, pain caused by movement is avoided; also while the range of motion is being increased, muscle strength is being improved. If time is a factor, the PNF hold-relax procedure produces better results in a shorter period of time. Passive

mobilization, or some other method of mobilization, however, may be necessary when the patient is uncooperative or lacks voluntary control.

SUMMARY

49. Thirty subjects were studied to compare the effects of PNF hold-relax and passive mobilization on tight hamstring muscles. All subjects were mobilized for three weeks followed by one week without mobilization. Statistical analysis of the data showed the PNF hold-relax procedure to be more effective in increasing the range of motion of shortened tissue than passive mobilization. Also, the increase in range occurred at a faster rate with the PNF hold-relax procedure than with passive mobilization.

ACKNOWLEDGMENT

David Hinkley, Ph.D., designed the parametric statistical analysis.

REFERENCES

1. Egli, H.: Basis for selection of mobilization techniques. Phys. Ther. Rev. 38:759, 1957.
2. Knott, M., and Voss, D. E.: Proprioceptive Neuromuscular Facilitation, ed. 2. Harper and Row, New York, 1968.
3. Brunnstrom, S.: Clinical Kinesiology, ed. 2. F. A. Davis Company, Philadelphia, 1966.
4. Kabat, H.: Studies on neuromuscular dysfunction XIII: New concepts and techniques of neuromuscular reeducation for paralysis. Permanente Foundation Medical Bulletin 8: No. 3, 1950.
5. Ruch, T. C., and Patton, H. D.: Physiology and Biophysics. W. B. Saunders Company, Philadelphia, 1965.
6. Guyton, A. C.: Textbook of Medical Physiology, ed. 3. W. B. Saunders Company, Philadelphia, 1965.
7. Houk, J., and Hennemann, E.: Responses of Golgi tendon organs to active contraction of the soleus muscle of the cat. J. Neurophysiol. 30:466, 1967.
8. Best, C. H., and Taylor, N. B.: The Physiological Basis of Medical Practice, ed. 8. The Williams & Wilkins Company, Baltimore, 1966.
9. Levine, M. G., et al.: Relaxation of spasticity by physiological techniques. Arch. Phys. Med. 35:214, 1954.
10. Adams, A.: Effects of various conditioning programs on ligament strength. Southwest District AAHPER Convention, 1965.

REDUCTION OF STRESS BETWEEN MOTHERS AND THEIR HANDICAPPED CHILDREN*

Nancy B. Tyler and Kate L. Kogan

This paper reports the results of videotaped baselines and a series of behavioral instruction sessions that involved 18 preschool handicapped children and their mothers. The behaviors of mother and child were analyzed from videotaped records before, immediately following, and nine months after the behavioral instruction sessions. The intervention, the instruction sessions, focused on enrichment of the mother-child interaction repertoire and was accomplished with immediate feedback to the mother by using the "bug-in-the-ear" device. The frequencies of the 216 measures of negative behaviors tested (12 behaviors in each of 18 dyads) decreased in 48 instances immediately following the instruction sessions. Forty of these changes were still present nine months later. The research indicates it is possible to reduce stressful, negative interaction and, in addition, to maintain the mother's behaviors of warmth and acceptance.

1.   The concept that child behaviors have a measurable effect on their parents' behavior[1, 2] is an important idea when considering specific

---

*Reprinted with permission of the American Occupational Therapy Association, Inc., from the *American Journal of Occupational Therapy* 31:151–155, 1977.

home treatment program for parents of handicapped children. The experience of parenting a handicapped child may impose certain kinds of structure and stress on parents' response styles that are qualitatively and quantitatively different from those experienced by parents of nonhandicapped children.[3, 4] In addition, parenting a delayed child may not give the mother the stimulation and positive feedback other children provide.

2. In a previous observation study, young cerebral-palsied children and their mothers were followed over a two-year period. The interactions that occurred while mother and child played together were compared with those that occurred while they were engaged in therapy. The results demonstrated that, when mothers were performing therapy, both mother and child displayed greater amounts of negative behaviors than when they were playing, and that mothers became excessively controlling.[5] These behaviors persisted over the two-year period.[6] In addition, there was a progressive reduction of the warm and positive behaviors in play and therapy sessions.[7] This decrease in behaviors such as smiling, positive verbal statements, and physical closeness was termed "affect turn-off."

3. Mothers were often preoccupied about their ability to position the child's limbs properly at the expense of the child's comfort or satisfaction. Also, they frequently seemed to view the child's inability to perform as a demonstration of their own inadequacy in working with him or her. Mothers were likely to be so intent on achieving the desired goal that they repeatedly called the child's errors to the child's attention, and often failed to support the child's less-than-successful efforts to comply. Mothers tended to be determined to continue with a frustrating activity long after the child became irritable and uncooperative, and on occasion they forbade the child to play with the attractive toys in the room so that a particular exercise could be completed.

4. On the basis of these findings it seemed important that mothers acquire more positive and rewarding attitudes toward the child, become more comfortable in interacting with their child, augment their interactive repertoires while they integrated therapy into play activities, and modify the interpersonal climate in which mother and child were communicating.

5. The present study reports the results of an observation-intervention program with preschool handicapped children and their mothers. At the outset the following hypotheses were stated:

1. Observational records and their analyses will reveal a greater incidence of stressful and conflicted interactions between mother and

child during therapy before the mother's behavioral instruction series than afterward.

2. Mothers who have been taught specific ways of interacting with their children will persist in displaying those interaction styles over a period of time after the instruction series has ended.

6.   An additional goal of the research was to prevent the gradual occurrence of "affect turn-off." It was anticipated that helping the mothers acquire and maintain more positive and warm behaviors toward their children would indicate a more comfortable interaction.

METHODS

Subjects

7.   The study involved 18 children and their mothers. The group contained 11 boys and 7 girls ranging in age from 21 to 61 months, all attending the Children's Clinic and Preschool in Seattle. Fifteen children were diagnosed as having cerebral palsy; 3 were identified as developmentally delayed with generalized hypotonia. The motor skills impairment of the group ranged from two children with almost no head, trunk, or extremity control, to a 33-month-old mild hemiplegic who had acquired most of the motor skills expected of a child that age. Developmental ages, measured by the Bayley Scales of Infant Development,[8] ranged from a child who scored below the two-month level to three children whose skills exceeded the two and one-half year ceiling of the scale. The mothers as subjects were not selected according to age, educational level, socioeconomic status, family size, or constellation. Therefore, these factors covered a wide range.

8.   All children received individual therapy from an occupational or physical therapist trained in the neurodevelopmental approach. Some parent instruction was included and, in addition, some children participated in a classroom or speech therapy or both. Therapists and teachers referred children to the project when a mother-child conflict was apparent or when the parent expressed interest in the study project. The staff therapist participated with the research staff in the weekly behavioral instruction series with each mother and child. The child's school and therapy program continued unaltered.

Procedure

9.   All baseline videorecordings and the behavioral instruction sessions took place in a room in the preschool. Sessions were observed and

video-taped through a one-way mirror from an adjacent room. The child's therapist helped to select toys and therapy equipment that were functionally appropriate for each child. The selected toys and equipment were presented to the mother and child on each of their baseline observations in order to standardize the situation for that particular dyad.

10.   Two 42-minute sessions in which the mother was instructed to "play and do therapy" were videorecorded a week apart (Time 1). The videotapes provided a baseline record of the recurrent interaction style of a particular mother-child pair. Selected samples of the videotape were then reviewed with the mother. Areas of behaviors that the mothers viewed as problems were discussed, and an effort was made to relate the videotaped observations to the problem areas. The joint information thus derived was translated into specific behavioral suggestions for the mother to follow in the playroom during the weekly behavioral instruction sessions. Videotaped segments were identified as examples of interactions that ought to be encouraged and interactions that ought to be discouraged. The mother practiced these behaviors for eight weeks in half-hour play and therapy sessions during which she wore a "bug-in-the-ear" that permitted the observer to provide her with behavioral instructions from the adjacent room. The observer acknowledged when the mother carried out suggestions successfully, suggested further opportunities for her to use desired behaviors, and commented on specific things she might do or say. The behavioral instruction series was conducted by a two-member team. One member was from the project staff and the other was a staff therapist from the clinic—when possible, the child's regular therapist. Follow-up videotaped data was collected immediately following the eight instruction sessions (Time 2) and nine months later (Time 3, or one year after the initial baselines).

Analysis

11.   The videotaped behavior records were analyzed by using the Interpersonal Behavior Constructs[9] system. This system consists of a checklist of behavior transactions identified in past research and clinical experience as representing a range of important interactions. The transactions characterize the unique interpersonal styles of a wide variety of mother-child dyads. Behavior observations are analyzed in 40-second time units.

12.   The content of the checklist items falls into the following groups of categories. The focus of each participant's *attention* is identified as being primarily on the activity of the other person, on the participant's

264

own activity, or on joint activity. *Vocalization* is classified as being absent or limited, one-sided, or reciprocal and related. *Lead taking* is assessed in terms of recurrent attempts to impose structure on the other person's behavior whether engaged in individual or joint activity. These behaviors are checked only if their duration characterizes the major portion of the 40-second time unit being reviewed.

13.   The remainder of the items are viewed as being important even if they occur only once during the 40-second time interval being assessed. One cluster of items covers specific instances of *positive behaviors*—smiling, animated voice, stating personal pleasure, physical closeness, or expression of affection. Another section of the list itemizes behaviors that imply *negative feelings*. Pouting, frowning, and tone of voice are checked here. Note is made of slaps, snatches, threat-gestures or other aggressive acts toward the other person or the thing with which the person is occupied. Note is also made of ambiguous affect such as that reflected in sarcasm. A group of items reflects various manifestations of efforts to *dominate* the other person's behavior—for example, criticizing or intruding physically into the other person's activity. Another group of items covers behaviors that reflect a variety of *submissive* roles, such as seeking permission, or activity complying with the other person's direction. A final listing was made of the mother's physical repositioning or holding the child in a therapy position.

RESULTS

14.   An earlier longitudinal study[7] employed a system of behavioral analysis, Interpersonal Behavior Ratings, that served to identify stressful interpersonal behaviors as those that included elements of strong control, or negative affect, or both. Prior to the beginning of the present study the videotape assessment procedures were revised into the Interpersonal Behavior Constructs format.[9] On the basis of a correlational analysis of the two systems, the following items of the revised system were identified as constituting stress indicators: *Mother Control, Mother Lead, Mother Negative Content, Child Negative Content, Mother Negative Voice, Child Negative Voice, Mother Mixed Message, Child Mixed Message, Mother Physical Hostility, Child Physical Hostility, Mother Intrusion,* and *Child Intrusion.* Initially, no single mother-child dyad exhibited all of the stressful behaviors. Each dyad revealed one or several of the negative behaviors listed.

15.   The method of analysis is based on 126 time units for each dyad in each set of two videorecordings. A nested analysis of variance pro-

cedure permits comparison of a single pair's scores at the three time points: preintervention (Time 1), immediately after the instruction series (Time 2), and nine months later (Time 3). Thus, researchers test whether or not the difference in the rate of occurrence of a particular behavior at the different time points is systematically greater than chance differences, or than random differences between the subsections of any given single session. The data from each mother-child pair are treated individually so that each pair serves as its own control.

16. Some reductions of negative behaviors were found in 14 of the 18 dyads. There were 216 measures tested (12 negative behaviors $\times$ 18 dyads). Since each mother-child pair had only a few of the stressful behaviors at the outset, there was no expectation that any dyad would exhibit more than a few changes. Between Time 1 (initial baseline observations) and Time 2 (baseline observations immediately following behavior instruction series), the 18 mother-child pairs exhibited decreases in 48 of the 216 measures tested.

17. At Time 3, 12 months after initial baselines, 40 of the 48 changes tabulated above were still present to a statistically significant degree ($p \leq .01$). There were seven additional instances of decrease that had not been in evidence at Time 2. Table 1 details these findings.

18. Four other behavior changes in the direction opposite to that predicted occurred between Time 2 and Time 3. Thirteen of the 18 mother-child dyads accounted for the decreases that persisted over the course of the study. Thus the two hypotheses were confirmed.

19. The goal of the intervention procedure was not only to reduce the incidence of stressful interactions, but also to prevent the gradual occurrence of "affect turn-off." The following Interpersonal Behavior Construct items refer to warmth and acceptance: *Mother Smiles, Enthusiasm, Mother Praise,* and *Mother Physical Warmth.* According to the Wilcoxon Matched-pairs, Signed-ranks Test, none of these behaviors decreased significantly for the group over the one-year period between Time 1 and Time 3. When the observation records of individual mother-child dyads were examined singly, one mother exhibited significantly less *Praise* at the end of the study than she had at the beginning (according to an analysis of variance); no other significant decreases in warmth or acceptance were noted in any of the other mothers.

DISCUSSION

20. The findings show that it was possible to reduce stressful and conflicted interactions through an eight-week series of personalized

Table 1. Changes in negative behaviors (Time 1 vs. Time 3)

Subjects	A	B	C	D	E	F	G	H	I	J	K	L	M	N	O	P	Q	R	
Mother Control	*	*	D	*	*	*	*	*	—		*		*	X			D		11
Mother Lead	*	*	*	*	*	*	*	—			*	—	D	X					9
Mother Negative Content		*	*	*	*	*			—	D				*					7
Child Negative Content	—		*					X	—										1
Mother Negative Voice	*		*																2
Child Negative Voice	*		*	*	—					*									4
Mother Mixed Message	*	*	*																3
Child Mixed Message																			0
Mother Physical Hostility	*											X							1
Child Physical Hostility	*			*															2
Mother Intrusion	*	*	D	D	*														5
Child Intrusion	—	*								D									2
Final Decreases	8	6	8	6	4	3	2	1	0	3	2	0	2	1	0	0	1	0	47

*, Significant decreases at both 3 and 12 months after intial baselines.

—, Significant decreases at 3 months, not maintained at 12 months.

D, Significant decreases at 12 months.

X, Significant increases at 12 months.

behavioral instruction. More than four-fifths of the changes remained significant nine months after the instruction series ended.

21.   Most of the change was in mother behaviors, but 12 of the changes reflected less negative behaviors on the part of the child. This falls in line with one of the basic assumptions of the project: namely, that parents play an active role in their child's learning either adaptive or maladaptive behaviors. The focus of the study had been on the interaction *between* people rather than the particular behaviors of either individual. Thus, in accordance with the view that social interaction is a reciprocal process, the results demonstrated that by changing one element in the dyadic relationship, the other element also changed.

22.   There was no evidence of gradual "affect turn-off" in this sample of mothers of young cerebral-palsied children, drawn from the same treatment facility (though at a later date) as the mothers who had exhibited "affect turn-off" in the earlier study. The evidence implied that the mother-instruction series had helped to avert any decrement in expressions of positive feeling. Michelman[10] suggests that a child's play is crucial to the development of behavior, thinking, and performance. The pediatric occupational therapist may guide the parents of a child with deficits in being an attentive audience and enjoying their child's play.

23.   The extent to which social interaction depends on normal development is often overlooked. The nonhandicapped child's growth and

development in the first two years is rapid, positive, and covers many facets. Interaction skills develop quickly with facial, gestural, and vocal components. There is a rapid move toward independence, mobility, expression of ideas and desires, self-help skills, and self-initiated play. Normal children elicit positive interaction not only from their parents, but also from many other adults in their environment. Thus, parents can derive satisfaction from their child's development and behaviors. In contrast, parents of physically handicapped children face slow progress. The parents may expend energy, time, and money on a situation that seems nonresponsive to their efforts. As the mother of a handicapped child tends to that child's needs, time for her other children, her spouse, and her own social and self-improvement is limited.

24. Viewing this situation from a wider vantage point, therapists may ask whether or not mothers of severely handicapped children need to maintain their own mental health over time by altering some of their interactions with the child. One way for a mother to cope with her problems is to disengage herself increasingly from her child. It is probable that the "affect turn-off" documented in the previous study was one form of disengagement. A mother's disengagement from her child would be healthier for both mother and child if it were in the context of reducing the quantity of involvement with her child, rather than of reducing its quality.

25. In other words, mothers might be urged to maintain an active and positive interaction, but to decrease the time spent with the handicapped child. In essence, this is the experience most parents have in raising children. As nonhandicapped preschool and school-aged children acquire skills and independence, they spend less time with their parents. The *quality*, rather than the quantity, of the interaction between the mother and child appears to be the important factor.

26. The results of this research suggest that physically handicapped children have a more difficult time participating in reciprocal interaction, especially in a positive or active way; and thus the mother is "stuck" in interaction that does not proceed at the rapid rate exhibited by a nonhandicapped child, and that is not as rewarding.

27. Pediatric occupational therapists engaged in working with physically handicapped children and their parents have frequently encountered difficulty in enlisting parent cooperation in activities designed to facilitate the child's growth and development. Although a variety of methods have been contrived to involve the parent in the process, gaps have remained between the professional's recommendations and the parent's ability to carry them out. Current emphasis has been on teaching parents to be therapists. Because this may be an in-

trusion into the parent role, the therapist needs to focus on *guiding* parents toward a healthy interaction with their child. The results of this research may provide some clues to the reasons for the professional-parent gap, and suggest new directions for parent guidance.

SUMMARY

28.   The slow development of the physically handicapped youngster has an effect on the social interaction between a mother and her child. The results of an eight-week series of personalized behavioral instruction to the mothers of handicapped children showed that stressful interaction could be changed and the change maintained. The behavioral instructions were offered to 18 mothers; however, the altered behaviors that occurred in both the mothers and the children suggest a reciprocal nature in social interactions. By changing one element in the dyadic relationship, the other element was also changed. In addition, the mothers maintained expressions of positive affect throughout the study that suggests the mother's role as an attentive audience and in enjoying the child's play can be important components of the interaction.

ACKNOWLEDGMENT

This study was supported by Grant MC-R-530248 from the Bureau of Community Health Services, Maternal and Child Health and Crippled Children's Services, U.S. Department of Health, Education and Welfare.

REFERENCES

1. Bell, R. Q.: A reinterpretation of the direction of effects in studies of socialization. Psychol. Rev. 75:81, 1968.
2. Beckwith, L.: Relationships between infants' social behavior and their mothers' behaviors. Child. Dev. 43:397, 1972.
3. Marshall, N. R., et al.: Verbal Interactions: Mothers and their retarded children vs. mothers and their non-retarded children. Am. J. Ment. Defic. 77:415, 1973.
4. O'Conner, W. A., and Stachowiak, J. G.: Patterns of Interaction in families with low adjusted, high adjusted and mentally retarded members. Family Process 10:229, 1971.
5. Tyler, N. B., and Kogan, K. L.: The social by-products of therapy with young children. Phys. Ther. 52:508, 1972.
6. Tyler, N. B., et al.: Interpersonal components of therapy with young cerebral palsied. Am. J. Occup. Ther. 28:395, 1974.
7. Kogan, K. L., et al.: The process of interpersonal adaptation between mothers and their cerebral palsied children. Dev. Med. Child. Neurol. 16:518, 1974.

8. Bayley, N.: Bayley Scales of Infant Development. The Psychological Corporation, New York, 1969.
9. Kogan, K. L., and Gordon, B. N.: Interpersonal behavior constructs: A revised approach to defining dyadic interaction styles. Psychol. Rep. 36:835, 1975.
10. Michelman, S. S.: Play and the deficit child. In Reilly, M. (ed.): Play as Exploratory Learning. Sage Publications, Beverly Hills, 1974, pp. 157–207.

INDEX

274